Examinat...
Nerve Inj...

An Anatomical Appro...

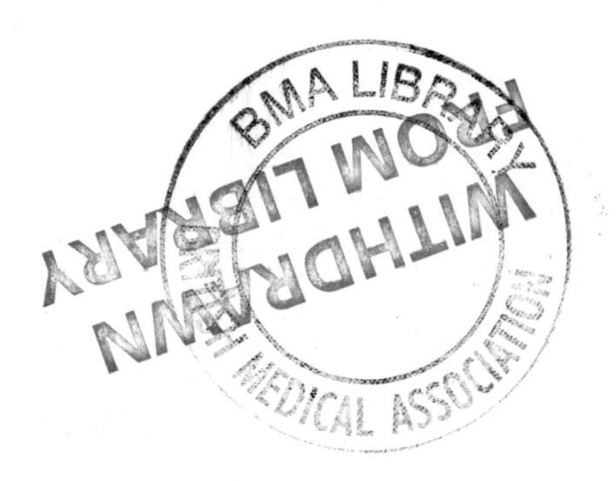

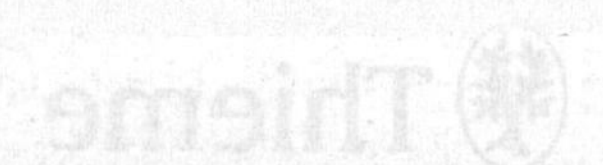

Examination of Peripheral Nerve Injuries

An Anatomical Approach

Stephen M. Russell, M.D.
Assistant Professor
Department of Neurosurgery
New York University School of Medicine
New York, New York

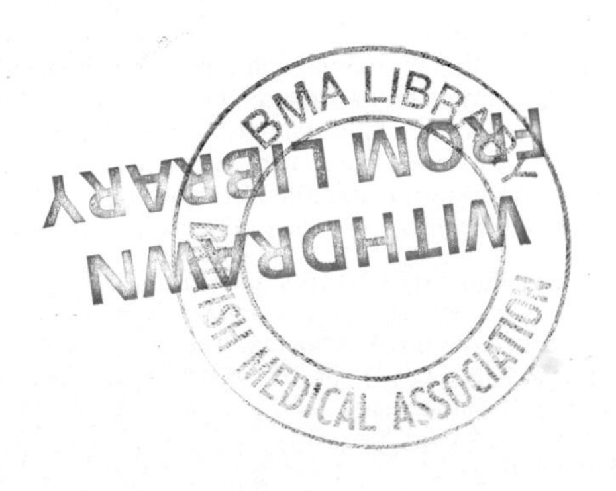

Thieme
New York • Stuttgart

Thieme Medical Publishers, Inc.
333 Seventh Ave.
New York, NY 10001

Library of Congress Cataloging-in-Publication Data
Russell, Stephen M.
Examination of peripheral nerve injuries: an anatomical approach / Stephen M. Russell.
p. ; cm.
Includes bibliographical references and index.
ISBN-13: 978-1-58890-483-6 (alk. paper)
ISBN-10: 1-58890-483-0 (alk. paper)
ISBN-13: 978-3-13-143071-7 (alk. paper)
ISBN-10: 3-13-143071-0 (alk. paper)
1. Nerves, Peripheral—Wounds and injuries. I. Title. [DNLM: 1. Peripheral Nerves—anatomy & histology. 2. Peripheral Nerves—injuries. 3. Nervous System Diseases—diagnosis. WL 500 R967e 2006]

RD595.R87 2006
617.4'83–dc22 2006013881

Important note: Medical knowledge is ever-changing. As new research and clinical experience broaden our knowledge, changes in treatment and drug therapy may be required. The authors and editors of the material herein have consulted sources believed to be reliable in their efforts to provide information that is complete and in accord with the standards accepted at the time of publication. However, in view of the possibility of human error by the authors, editors, or publisher of the work herein or changes in medical knowledge, neither the authors, editors, nor publisher, nor any other party who has been involved in the preparation of this work, warrants that the information contained herein is in every respect accurate or complete, and they are not responsible for any errors or omissions or for the results obtained from use of such information. Readers are encouraged to confirm the information contained herein with other sources. For example, readers are advised to check the product information sheet included in the package of each drug they plan to administer to be certain that the information contained in this publication is accurate and that changes have not been made in the recommended dose or in the contraindications for administration. This recommendation is of particular importance in connection with new or infrequently used drugs.

Some of the product names, patents, and registered designs referred to in this book are in fact registered trademarks or proprietary names even though specific reference to this fact is not always made in the text. Therefore, the appearance of a name without designation as proprietary is not to be construed as a representation by the publisher that it is in the public domain.

Printed in China

5 4 3 2 1

TMP ISBN 978-1-58890-483-6
TMP ISBN 1-58890-483-0
GTV ISBN 978 3 13 143071 7
GTV ISBN 3-13-143071-0

I dedicate this work to S.A.H.

Contents

Foreword

There are few things in medicine and surgery that give as much personal satisfaction as a well-done physical examination, which can localize a lesion and often identify its nature. This is despite the fact that modern medicine includes a huge array of biochemical, imaging, and electrodiagnostic studies. The physical examination takes on special importance for the patient who has a peripheral neuropathy because although extremely valuable, imaging and electrodiagnostic studies only help to "color the picture." The original sketch has to include both the history and a careful physical examination. A common mistaken perception is that the electromyogram (EMG) and conduction studies can replace the clinical motor and sensory examination. This is not the case at all; indeed, a good EMG technician always examines the limb or portion of the body in question before doing the electrical study.

Articles, textbooks, and monographs such as the *MRC Handbook* have been published but there has not been enough emphasis on the mechanics of the examination. Dr. Russell has provided this as well as an accurate account of the anatomy of each major nerve and its branches. He ably systematizes the examination for each nerve, including the brachial and pelvic plexuses, based on the concept that nerves tend to innervate muscles in a cascade-like fashion. When the examination steps documented in this text are mastered, then entities such as Martin–Gruber anastomosis or the anterior interosseous syndrome become easier to understand as well as remember.

In addition, Dr. Russell gives useful insights about various nerve injuries and entrapments and the syndromes relating to them. This information is especially detailed in the chapters on upper-extremity nerves. Throughout the book, the well-selected and detailed figures provide an excellent compliment to the text.

The reader will enjoy perusing as well as a more careful study of *The Examination of Peripheral Nerve Injury: An Anatomical Approach*. It is a welcome addition to the neurological literature.

David G. Kline, M.D.
Boyd Professor
Louisiana State University Health Science Center

Preface

After completing my residency in neurological surgery, I decided to study the diagnosis and surgical management of peripheral nerve disorders. In preparation for this training, however, I realized there were few books available that specifically provided instruction on how to examine patients with focal peripheral neuropathies. I found this surprising, considering the frequency with which these problems occur in clinical practice.

Recognizing the need for such a text, I collected my notes and experiences during my peripheral nerve fellowship and organized them into a book that teaches the reader how to examine a patient with a suspected focal neuropathy. This approach includes the pertinent anatomy of each peripheral nerve, photographs illustrating muscular examination techniques, and discussions regarding localization and diagnosis. Because a strong understanding of anatomical relationships is paramount for examining patients with nerve injury, this is stressed throughout the book.

Numerous and confusing anatomical variations are commonplace in the peripheral nervous system, which makes absorbing this anatomy difficult. Therefore, in this book I concentrate only on the most common variations, using both schematic figures and simplified text descriptions to facilitate learning. Less common variations, which are nonetheless important, are discretely placed in the text and are highlighted in bold with a diamond at the beginning of the note. Some anatomical variations and alternative muscular examination techniques have been omitted for simplicity.

This monograph has eight chapters. It begins with a discussion of the three major peripheral nerves of the upper extremity: the median, ulnar, and radial nerves. These nerves are discussed first so the proximal brachial plexus can be described in the context of these distal extremity branches, simplifying this very complicated and intimidating structure. The discussion of the brachial plexus is split into two chapters. The first reviews anatomy and the examination of muscles innervated by its smaller branches; the second discusses the overall approach to brachial plexus injury localization and diagnosis. The last three chapters address the lower extremities, an aspect of peripheral nerve diagnosis often abbreviated in other texts. The lower extremity is discussed as thoroughly as the upper. The major lower-extremity nerves are similarly reviewed first, so the discussion of the lumbosacral plexus in the final chapter makes more sense.

Peripheral nerve entrapment and injury are common, and encountered by most medical professionals on a daily basis. I hope this book makes the examination and diagnosis of these injuries more understandable for all.

Acknowledgments

I thank Dr. David Kline for teaching me, and countless others how to properly examine patients with peripheral nerve injury.

I would also like to acknowledge the following physicians who each contributed to my peripheral nerve training, and therefore to the creation of this book: Robert Tiel, Patrick Kelly, David Chiu Kartik Krishnan, Rashid Janjua, Paul Pannu, Linda Yang, Susan Durham, Michael Strupp, Hans Peter Richter, Gregor Antoniadis, Hans Assmus, Thomas Dombert, and Mario Siqueira.

I would like to acknowledge the authors of several books on peripheral nerve diagnosis and surgery that I read during my fellowship, because much of the factual information and figures in my book merely represent a summary or simplification of these more comprehensive and scientific publications. They include: *Focal Peripheral Neuropathies* by John Stewart, *Nerve Injuries: Operative Results for Major Nerve Injuries, Entrapments, and Tumors* by David Kline and Alan Hudson, *Surgery of the Peripheral Nerve* by Susan Mackinnon and Lee Dellon, *Operative Nerve Repair and Reconstruction* by Richard Gelberman, *Peripheral Nerve Lesions*

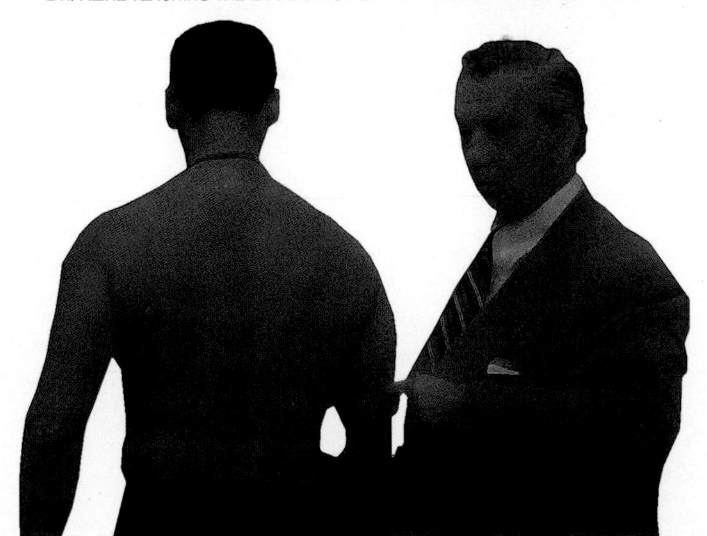

DR. KLINE TEACHING THE EXAMINATION OF PERIPHERAL NERVE INJURY - 2005

by G. Penkert and H. Fansa, *Nerve Injury and Repair* by Goran Lundborg, and the excellent illustrations in *Peripheral Neurology: Case Studies* by Jay Liveson.

I thank Ryan Kelley and David Chung for helping create the photographic images. I am indebted to those who kindly reviewed portions of this monograph for content and readability: Linda Yang, Nicholas Post, Emily Ridgeway, Kartik Krishnan, Rashid Jinjua, Erik Parker, and especially Sigrid Hahn.

This monograph was completed, in part, during my time as the 2004 Van Wagenen Fellow, and therefore I would like to thank the American Association of Neurological Surgeons as well as the Van Wagenen family for making this possible.

1

The Diagnostic Anatomy of the Median Nerve

The median nerve has contributions from four nerve roots via the brachial plexus (C6 to T1), and maintains a "median" location throughout its anatomical course down the upper extremity; whether along the intermuscular septum between the biceps and triceps, in the antecubital fossa, or distally at the wrist—the median nerve is always in the anatomical "center." From a functional standpoint, this nerve innervates key muscles of the hand, including those responsible for wrist flexion and movement of the first three fingers. Compression of the median nerve at the wrist results in carpal tunnel syndrome, the most common peripheral nerve entrapment seen in clinical practice.

♦ Anatomical Course

The Arm

The median nerve is derived from both the lateral and medial cords of the brachial plexus, with the lateral cord providing mostly sensory axons from C6 and C7, and the medial cord providing motor axons from C8 and T1. Therefore, the majority of motor input is from the medial cord. Based on their relationship to the axillary artery deep to the pectoralis minor muscle, the brachial plexus cords receive their names (medial, lateral, and posterior). In agreement with this nomenclature, when viewing the upper arm from its medial (inside) surface toward the axilla, the medial cord is medial to the axillary artery and the lateral cord is lateral to the axillary artery. Terminal divisions of the medial and lateral cords merge to create the median nerve, forming a Y-shaped confluence over the superficial surface of the brachial artery. Once formed, the median nerve travels distally while maintaining an intimate relationship with this artery in the upper arm.

The median nerve remains slightly lateral and superficial to the brachial artery as it passes down the arm. It runs anterior and parallel to the intermuscular septum, which separates the triceps from the arm flexors (i.e., biceps brachii, brachialis) (**Fig. 1–1**). When the inside of the upper arm is viewed from a medial viewpoint (e.g., with the arm abducted and externally rotated), the median nerve runs down the midline toward the antecubital fossa. About halfway down the arm, the median nerve crosses over the top of the brachial artery and then rests just medial to it by the time it passes under the bicipital aponeurosis (lacertus

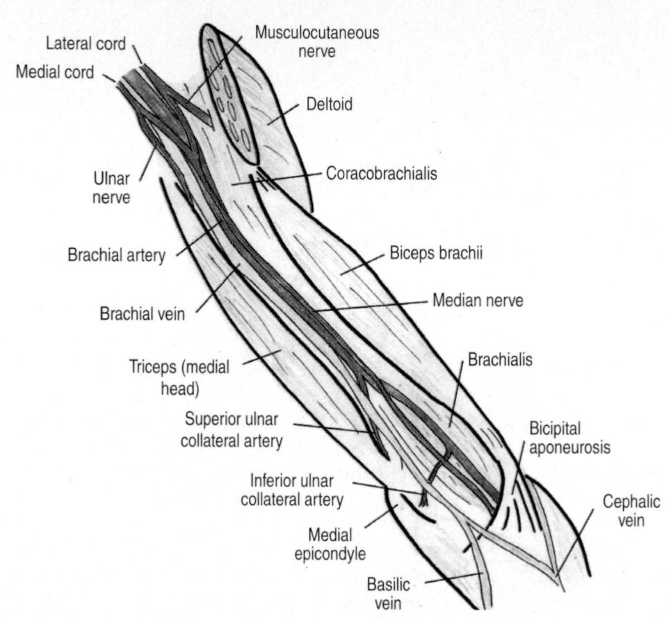

Figure 1–1 Median nerve in upper arm. The median nerve remains slightly lateral and superficial to the brachial artery as it passes down the arm. About halfway down the arm, the median nerve crosses over the top of the brachial artery and then rests just medial to it by the time it passes under the bicipital aponeurosis.

fibrosis) in the proximal forearm. The median nerve innervates no muscles in the arm, and in general, has no branches.

- **A few anatomical variations of the median nerve can occur in the arm. First, the medial and lateral cord components, which form the median nerve, may not fuse in the axilla, but instead join at various points along the arm, sometimes as low as the elbow. Second, these components may alternatively loop under the axillary/brachial artery, rather than superficial to it, when joining to form the median nerve. Finally, in some persons, the lateral component of the median nerve from the lateral cord is very small, with the majority of the median nerve's C6 and C7 fibers running instead in the musculocutaneous nerve, only to be returned to the median nerve via a communication about halfway down the arm. This temporary misrouting of innervation is not an uncommon phenomenon; it is almost as if the fibers took a wrong turn during development, asked for some directions, and rerouted themselves.**

The Antecubital Fossa/Elbow

At the elbow, the anatomy of the median nerve becomes more complex. It enters the antecubital fossa medial to the biceps brachii, passing over the brachialis muscle, which separates the nerve from the distal humerus. In the antecubital fossa, the median nerve passes under three successive arches or tunnels, bringing it deep into the forearm, only for it to re-emerge in the distal forearm prior to reaching the hand (**Fig. 1–2**). The first arch it passes under is the bicipital aponeurosis

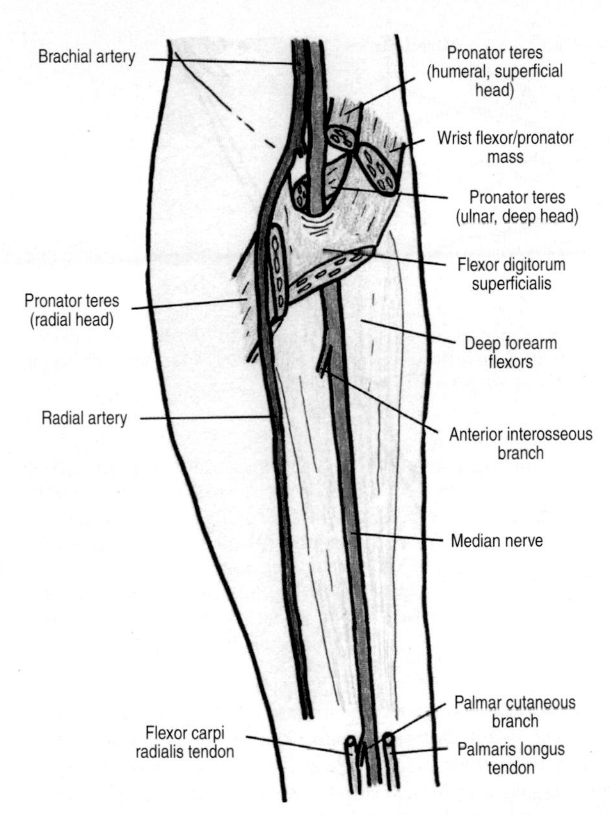

Figure 1–2 Median nerve in the forearm. In the antecubital fossa, the median nerve passes under three successive arches or tunnels (bicipital aponeurosis, pronator teres, and flexor digitorum superficialis), bringing it deep into the forearm, only for it to re-emerge in the distal forearm prior to reaching the hand.

(lacertus fibrosis), which is a thick layer of fascia attaching the biceps brachii to the proximal forearm flexor mass. Of note, one may directly palpate the median nerve prior to its diving below this aponeurosis by palpating two fingerbreadths proximal, and two lateral, to the medial epicondyle. Under this aponeurosis, the biceps tendon and brachial artery are both lateral, while the humeral head of the pronator teres muscle is medial to the median nerve (**Fig. 1–3**).

A short distance past the proximal edge of the bicipital aponeurosis, the median nerve dives below a second structure—the humeral head of the pronator teres. The pronator teres is a Y-shaped muscle with the bottom stem of the Y inserting into the radius distally and laterally. When viewing the antecubital fossa from anterior with the forearm supinated and extended, the Y of the pronator teres is turned on its side, so that the upper limbs of the Y are proximal, medial, and on top of each other. These proximal two heads include a larger superficial head that attaches to the humerus (humeral head), and a deeper, smaller head that attaches more distally to the ulna (ulnar head). The median nerve passes right in the crotch of this Y, with the ulnar head deep, and the humeral head superficial.

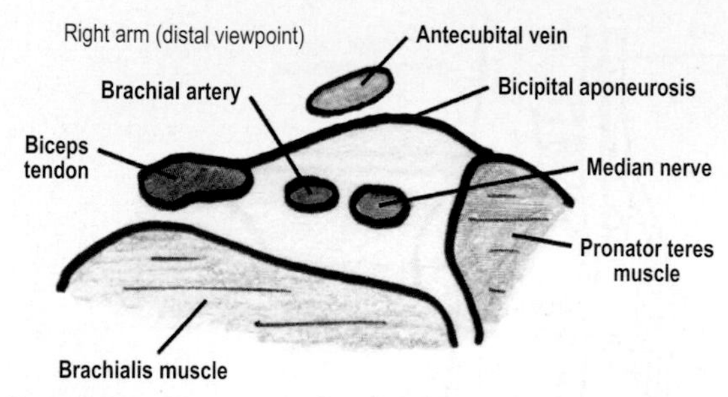

Figure 1–3 Cross section of median nerve in the antecubital fossa. The bicipital aponeurosis is superficial, the brachialis is deep, the biceps tendon and brachial artery are both lateral, and the humeral head of the pronator teres muscle is medial.

Next, just beyond the pronator teres, the median nerve almost immediately passes under a third structure: the two heads of the flexor digitorum superficialis (sublimis). This muscle's humeroulnar head is medial; its radial head is lateral. The flexor digitorum superficialis, in essence, forms a second Y through which the median nerve once again passes. In contrast to the pronator teres, however, when viewed anteriorly with the forearm supinated, the flexor digitorum superficialis' Y is not turned on its side. A fibrous ridge between its two heads is termed the *sublimis ridge,* and under this ridge, the median nerve passes.

◆ **Variations in this area are predominantly musculotendinous. Either the pronator teres or the flexor digitorum superficialis may have only one head, not two, and their proximal origins may vary. These muscular variations potentially create anatomical situations that may predispose to median nerve entrapment in the antecubital fossa.**

The Forearm

The median nerve travels down the center of the forearm deep to the digitorum superficialis, but superficial to the underlying flexor digitorum profundus. More precisely, the median nerve lies toward the lateral margin of the flexor digitorum profundus, near the flexor pollicis longus, which is the neighboring muscle on its lateral aspect. About one third or halfway down the forearm, an important branch of the median nerve, the *anterior interosseous nerve*, exits from its dorsolateral aspect. Once formed, the anterior interosseous nerve passes deeper in the forearm to run between the radius and ulna on the interosseous membrane, between and below the muscle bellies of the flexor digitorum profundus and flexor pollicis longus. This branch terminates in the distal forearm deep to the pronator quadratus. Near its origin, the anterior interosseus nerve passes under one or more fibrous ridges that originate off the pronator teres or flexor digitorum superficialis.

The median nerve proper continues down the arm, and becomes, once again, superficial about 5 cm proximal to the wrist crease, just medial to the flexor carpi radialis tendon. This muscle's tendon is the most prominent one that bowstrings proximal to the wrist (just lateral to midline) when the wrist is flexed against resistance. The palmaris longus tendon, when present, lies just medial to the median nerve at the proximal wrist. Once superficial, and before entering the hand, the median nerve gives a pure sensory branch, the *palmar cutaneous branch*, which runs superficial to the carpal tunnel and ramifies over the proximal, radial half of the palm, particularly over the thenar eminence. Occasionally, this sensory branch passes through its own tunnel in the transverse carpal ligament.

The brachial artery passes under the bicipital aponeurosis, where it bifurcates into the radial and ulnar arteries. The radial artery passes distally, near the superficial sensory radial nerve. The ulnar artery, alternatively, passes deep to the flexor-pronator mass, where it loops under the median nerve. In the distal forearm, the ulnar artery joins the ulnar nerve, and together they travel toward the wrist. Prior to passing below the median nerve in the antecubital fossa, the ulnar artery gives the interosseous communis artery, which shortly thereafter divides into the anterior and posterior interosseous arteries. The anterior interosseous artery passes distally with the anterior interosseous nerve, deep between the flexor pollicis longus and flexor digitorum profundus.

The Wrist/Hand

The median nerve passes through the center of the wrist in the carpal tunnel. A common analogy is to think of the carpal tunnel as an upside-down table. The tabletop is composed of carpal bones, with the legs of the table being the hook of the hamate and pisiform medially, and the tubercle of the trapezium and distal pole of the scaphoid laterally. Stretched over these legs, like a rug on an imaginary floor, is the thick transverse carpal ligament. From a volar viewpoint, the median nerve is the most superficial of nine structures running though the carpal tunnel. These other structures include the flexor pollicis longus tendon, four superficial flexor tendons, and four deep flexor tendons (**Fig. 1–4**). The palmaris longus tendon does not enter the carpal tunnel, but instead attaches more proximally to the superficially located palmaris aponeurosis. The flexor carpi radialis also does not pass through the carpal tunnel, but enters its own small tunnel, located lateral to the carpal tunnel, attaching to the second metacarpal bone.

After passing through the carpal tunnel, the median nerve gives a branch off its radial side: the *thenar motor branch* (or recurrent thenar motor branch). Then

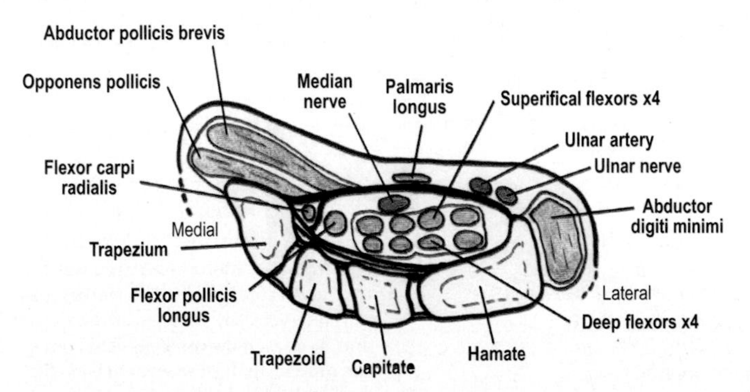

Figure 1–4 Cross section of median nerve in the carpal tunnel. From a volar viewpoint, the median nerve is the most superficial of nine structures running though the carpal tunnel. These other structures include the flexor pollicis longus tendon, four superficial flexor tendons, and four deep flexor tendons.

in the deep palm, the median nerve divides into two divisions, radial and ulnar. The radial division divides into the common digital nerve to the thumb, and the proper digital nerve to the radial half of the index finger. The common digital nerve to the thumb subsequently divides into the two proper digital nerves to the thumb. The ulnar division of the median nerve divides into the common digital nerves of the second and third web spaces, which also subsequently divide into proper digital nerves. The ulnar and radial divisions of the median nerve run deep (or dorsal) to the superficial palmar arch, but superficial to the flexor tendons.

- ♦ **Numerous variations in the origin and path of the thenar motor branch can occur. For instance, this motor branch may originate within the carpal tunnel, may pierce the transverse carpal ligament for a more direct route to the thenar muscles, and even emerge on the ulnar side of the median nerve, only to then cross deep or superficial to the median nerve to reach the thenar muscles. Other median nerve variations include (1) an early branching of the median nerve into radial and ulnar divisions proximal to the carpal tunnel (which often occurs with a "persistent median artery"), and (2) a connection between the thenar motor branch and the deep palmar branch of the ulnar nerve (discussed below).**

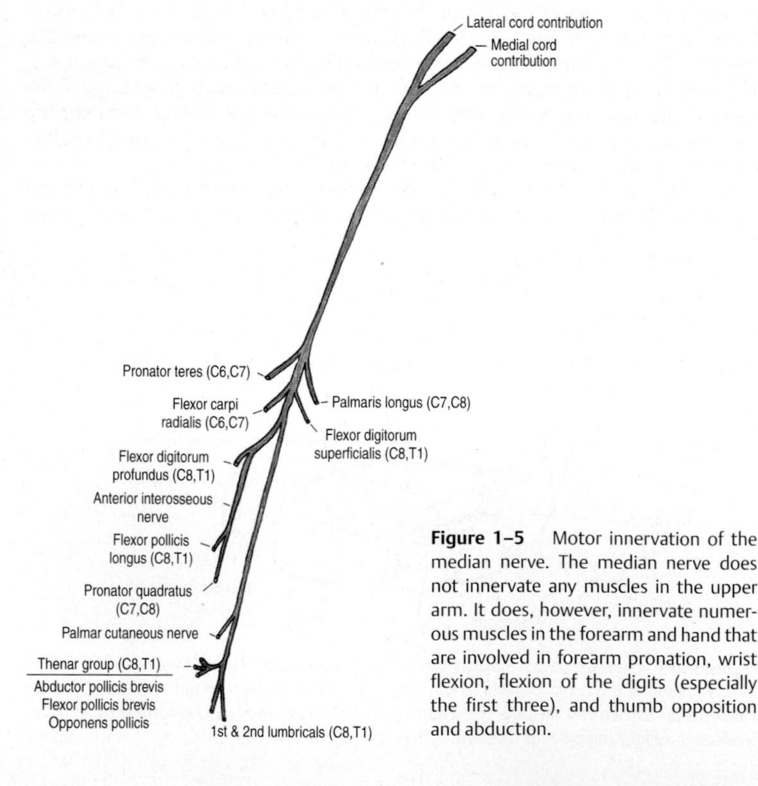

Figure 1–5 Motor innervation of the median nerve. The median nerve does not innervate any muscles in the upper arm. It does, however, innervate numerous muscles in the forearm and hand that are involved in forearm pronation, wrist flexion, flexion of the digits (especially the first three), and thumb opposition and abduction.

♦ Motor Innervation and Testing

The median nerve does not innervate any muscles in the upper arm. It does, however, innervate numerous muscles in the forearm and hand that are involved in forearm pronation, wrist flexion, flexion of the digits (especially the first three), and thumb opposition and abduction (**Fig. 1–5**). To aid memorization, these muscles may be separated into four sequential groups: proximal forearm, anterior interosseous, thenar motor, and terminal.

The Proximal Forearm Group

This group comprises four muscles: pronator teres, flexor carpi radialis, flexor digitorum superficialis, and palmaris longus. The *pronator teres* (C6, C7) is the main pronator of the forearm and the first muscle innervated by the median nerve. Branches to the pronator teres exit the median nerve at the lowest aspect of the upper arm, prior to the median nerve passing between the two heads of the pronator teres. From a mechanical perspective, the forearm needs to be extended for the pronator teres to have mechanical advantage. Therefore, to test this muscle the patient's forearm is first extended and then fully pronated. The patient is instructed to resist supination by the examiner (**Fig. 1–6**). The *flexor carpi radialis* (C6, C7) is one of the two major wrist flexors. The other is the *flexor carpi ulnaris*, which is innervated by the ulnar nerve. The flexor carpi radialis is the important wrist flexor, with loss of function severely limiting wrist flexion except in an ulnar direction. Test the flexor carpi radialis by having the patient flex the wrist along the trajectory of the forearm (**Fig. 1–7**). For severe weakness, have the patient flex the wrist with the forearm on a table, ulnar side down, which eliminates gravity. The tendon of the flexor carpi radialis can be seen and felt proximal to the wrist. The *palmaris longus* (C7, C8) is attached to the palmar aponeurosis and corrugates the palmar skin. This muscle is not readily examined for muscular strength, and in fact, is absent in about 15% of the population.

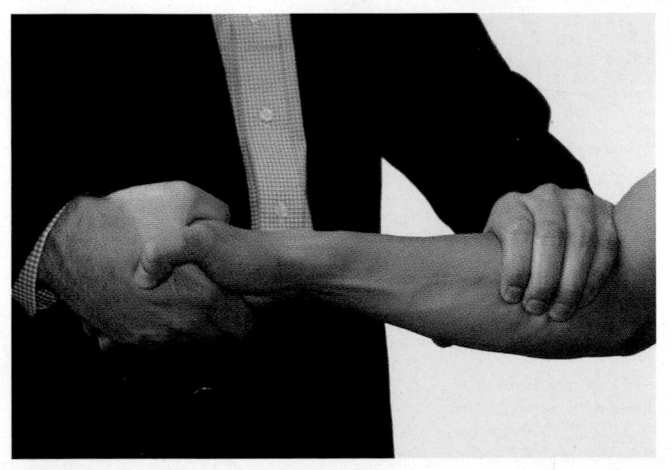

Figure 1–6 Pronator teres (C6, C7) assessment: The patient's forearm is extended and fully pronated. The patient is then instructed to resist supination of the forearm by the examiner.

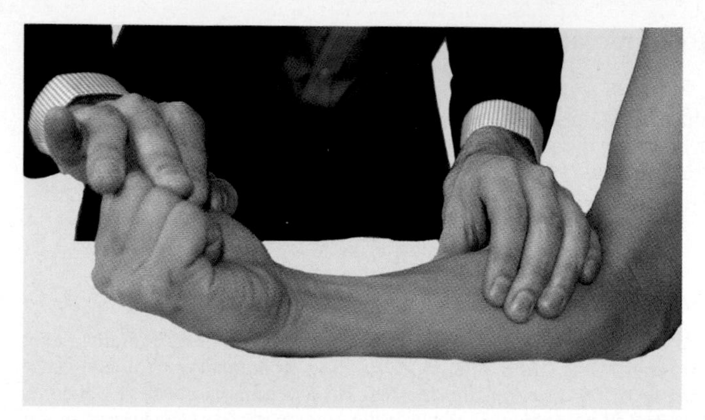

Figure 1–7 Flexor carpi radialis (C6, C7) assessment: The patient flexes the wrist along the trajectory of the forearm. For severe weakness, have the patient flex the wrist with the forearm on a table, ulnar side down, which eliminates gravity. Its tendon can be seen and felt proximal to the wrist.

The *flexor digitorum superficialis* (also known as the sublimis muscle, C8, T1) is also innervated by the median nerve and mediates flexion of the second to fifth digits (all except the thumb) at their proximal interphalangeal joints. To assess proximal interphalangeal joint flexion, each finger is tested separately. Placing your fingers between the patient's single finger to be tested and the remaining fingers isolates this movement (**Fig. 1–8**). This maneuver places the finger to be tested in mild flexion at the metacarpal–phalangeal (knuckle) joint, and simultaneously

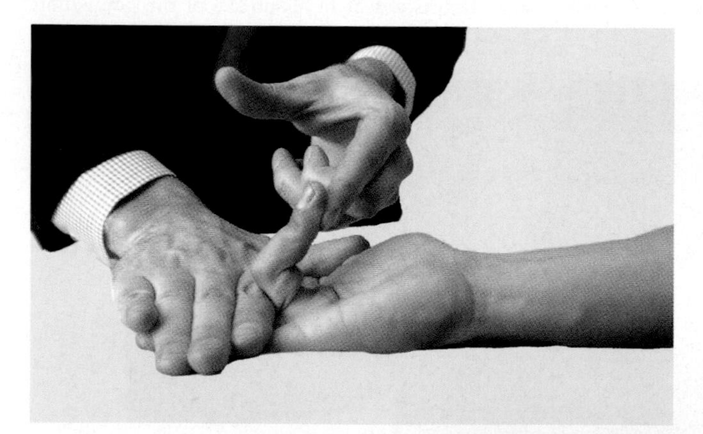

Figure 1–8 Flexor digitorum superficialis (C8, T1) assessment: To test proximal interphalangeal joint flexion, the supinated forearm and hand are placed straight. Each finger is tested separately. Placing your fingers between the single finger to be tested and the remaining fingers that are immobilized isolates this movement. This maneuver places the finger to be tested in mild flexion at the metacarpal–phalangeal (knuckle) joint, and stabilizes the remaining fingers in extension, a position that allows isolation of the flexor digitorum superficialis.

stabilizes the remaining fingers in extension, a position that allows isolation of the flexor digitorum superficialis.

A topographical aid in identifying the muscles of the medial forearm flexor mass is to place a hand on the opposite forearm with its thenar eminence on the medial epicondyle, the ring finger along the medial border of the forearm, and the rest of the fingers naturally lying over the forearm pointing in a distal trajectory toward the other hand. In this position, the thumb is over the pronator teres, the index finger is over the flexor carpi radialis, the long finger is over the palmaris longus, and the ring finger is along the flexor carpi ulnaris, the latter being innervated by the ulnar nerve.

- **In patients with pronator teres (and pronator quadratus, see below) weakness, a combination of arm abduction and internal rotation can allow gravity to mimic arm pronation. Furthermore, when testing pronation the patient should keep the fingers and hand relaxed to avoid substitution for pronation by the flexor carpi radialis and long finger flexors. When testing the finger flexors the wrist should be kept neutral and not allowed to extend because with wrist extension a tenodesis (distal joint movement mediated by lengthening the distance a tendon has to pass by changing the position of a more proximal joint) may occur that causes the fingers to passively flex.**

The Anterior Interosseous Group

This nerve innervates three deeply situated anterior forearm muscles: the flexor digitorum profundus (to the second and third digits), the flexor pollicis longus, and the pronator quadratus. The *flexor digitorum profundus* (C8, T1), as a whole, is innervated by both the median and ulnar nerves. The median nerve controls flexion of the distal interphalangeal joint of the second, and partly, the third digits; the ulnar nerve controls this muscle's action upon the third (partly), fourth, and fifth digits. Distal interphalangeal joint flexion of the third (or long) digit has

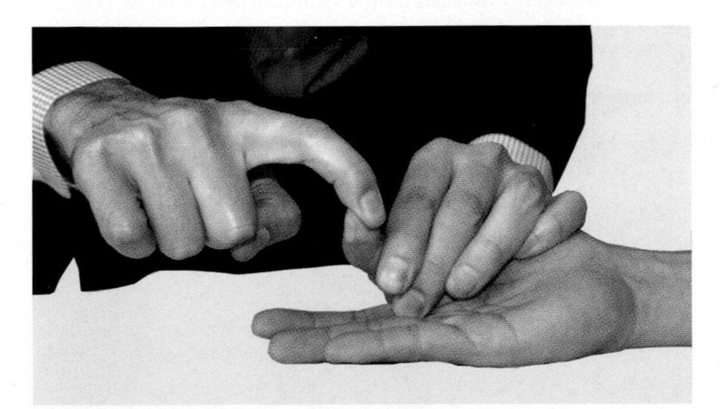

Figure 1–9 Flexor digitorum profundus (C8, T1) assessment: To assess the median innervation of the flexor digitorum profundus one should concentrate on the index finger. To do so, hold the metacarpal-phalangeal and proximal interphalangeal joints immobile, and have the patient flex the distal phalanx against your resistance.

variable dominance by the median or ulnar nerves. Additionally, even with complete denervation of one of these nerves, some movement of the long finger is usually preserved because both the median and ulnar portions of the flexor digitorum profundus act via a common tendon to this digit. Therefore, to assess in isolation median innervation of the flexor digitorum profundus one should concentrate on the index finger. To do so, hold the metacarpal-phalangeal and proximal interphalangeal joints immobile, and have the patient flex the distal phalanx against your resistance (**Fig. 1–9**). The *flexor pollicis longus* (C8, T1) performs a function similar to the profundus, but on the thumb; it flexes the distal phalanx of the thumb at the interphalangeal joint. Assess the flexor pollicis longus by immobilizing the thumb, except the interphalangeal joint, and ask the patient to flex the distal phalanx against resistance (**Fig. 1–10**). A quick way to assess both flexor digitorum profundus and flexor pollicis longus innervation from the anterior interosseous nerve is to ask the patient to make an okay sign by touching the tips of the thumb and index finger together. With weakness in these muscles, the distal phalanges cannot flex, and instead of the fingertips touching, the volar surfaces of each distal phalanx make contact (**Fig. 1–11**). The third muscle innervated by the anterior interosseous nerve is the *pronator quadratus* (C7, C8). This is a significantly weaker forearm pronator that the pronator teres. In fact, weakness in this muscle is often not readily apparent with a functioning pronator teres. However, with the forearm fully flexed, which removes the mechanical advantage of the pronator teres, weakness of the pronator quadratus should be detectable when compared with the normal arm. Test the pronator quadratus by having the patient resist supination of a fully flexed and pronated forearm (**Fig. 1–12**).

- **When testing the flexor digitorum profundus or the flexor pollicis longus, do not let the patient extend the distal interphalangeal joints prior to flexion because the passive re-flexion may mimic active joint flexion.**

The Thenar Group

The thenar group consists of three muscles innervated by the thenar motor branch of the median nerve. The first is the *abductor pollicis brevis* (C8, T1),

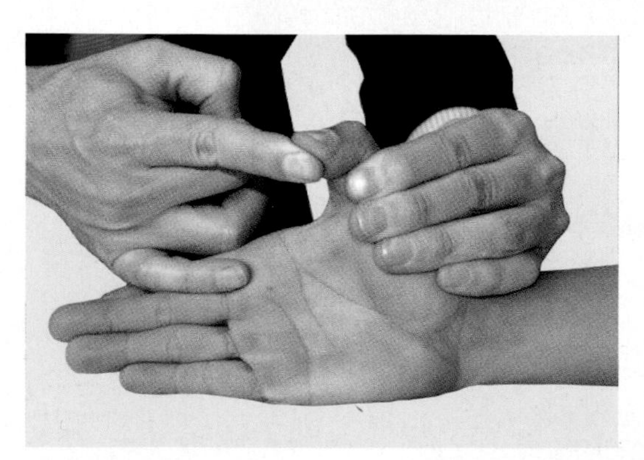

Figure 1–10 Flexor pollicis longus (C8, T1) assessment: Immobilize the thumb, except the interphalangeal joint, and then ask the patient to flex the distal phalanx against resistance.

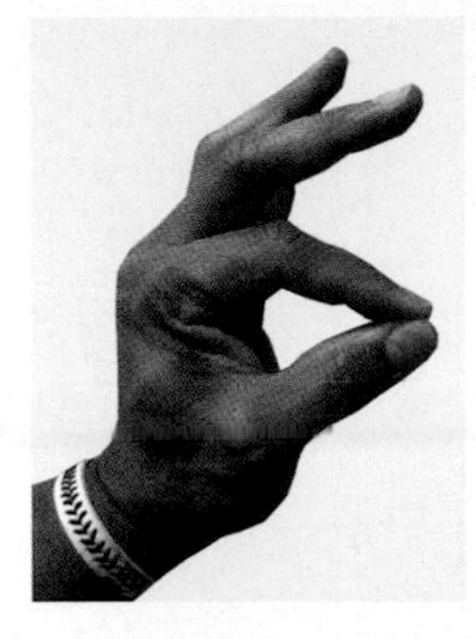

Figure 1–11 "Okay" or "circle" sign with anterior interosseous nerve weakness. A quick way to assess the flexor digitorum profundus and flexor pollicis longus innervation from the anterior interosseous nerve is to ask the patient to make an okay sign by touching the tips of the thumb and index finger together. With weakness in these muscles, the distal phalanges cannot flex, and instead of the fingertips touching, the volar surfaces of each distal phalanx make contact.

which as the name implies, abducts the thumb. Thumb abduction may be separated into two vectors: palmar abduction away from the plane of the palm (mediated by the abductor pollicis brevis), and radial abduction away from the line of the forearm (mediated by the abductor pollicis longus). Therefore, even

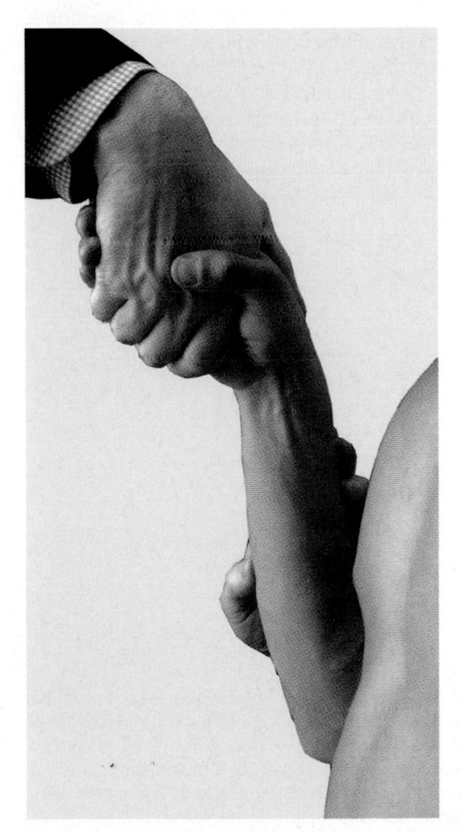

Figure 1–12 Pronator quadratus (C7, C8) assessment: Have the patient resist supination of a fully flexed and pronated forearm. With full forearm flexion, pronation by the usually dominant pronator teres is minimized.

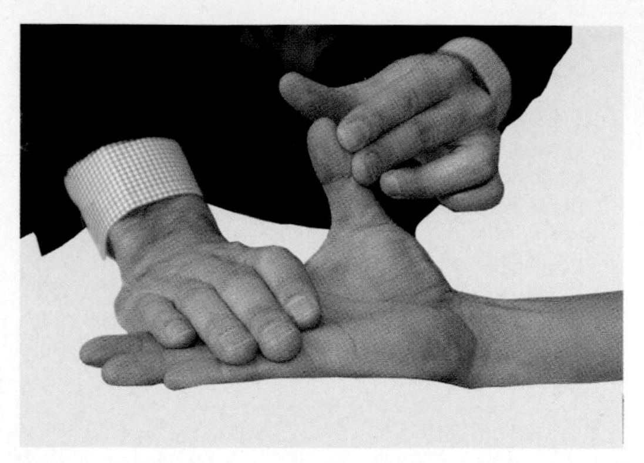

Figure 1–13 Abductor pollicis brevis (C8, T1) assessment: Resist movement of the thumb away from the plane of the palm (palmar abduction), while stabilizing the metacarpals of the remaining fingers.

with a complete palsy of the abductor pollicis brevis, radial abduction of the thumb can still occur. To test the abductor pollicis brevis, resist movement of the thumb away from the plane of the palm (palmar abduction) while the metacarpals of the remaining fingers are immobilized (**Fig. 1–13**). The *flexor pollicis brevis* (C8, T1) is innervated by both the median nerve (its superficial head) and ulnar nerve (its deep head). This muscle flexes the thumb at the metacarpal-phalangeal joint. To test the flexor pollicis brevis, immobilize the thumb's interphalangeal joint and have the patient flex at the metacarpal-phalangeal joint (**Fig. 1–14**). Make certain the distal interphalangeal joint does not flex because in allowing this,

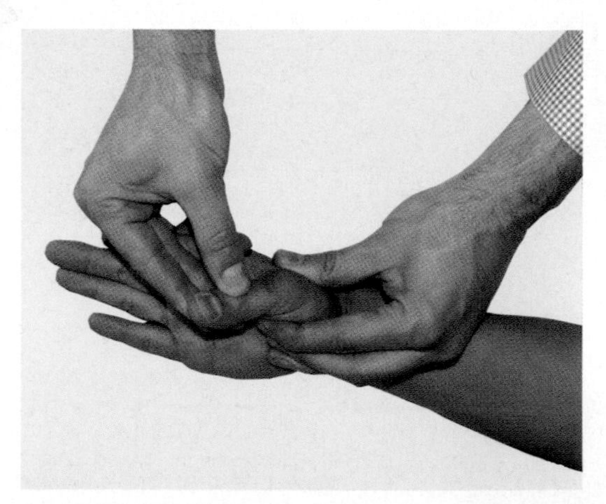

Figure 1–14 Flexor pollicis brevis (C8, T1) assessment: The patient flexes the thumb at the metacarpal-phalangeal joint against resistance placed over both the proximal and distal phalanges. Make certain the distal interphalangeal joint does not flex because in allowing this, substitution by the flexor pollicis longus occurs. Use your other hand to immobilize the first metacarpal to reduce substitution by the opponens pollicis. Because of its dual innervation, even with complete thenar motor branch palsies some thumb flexion still occurs.

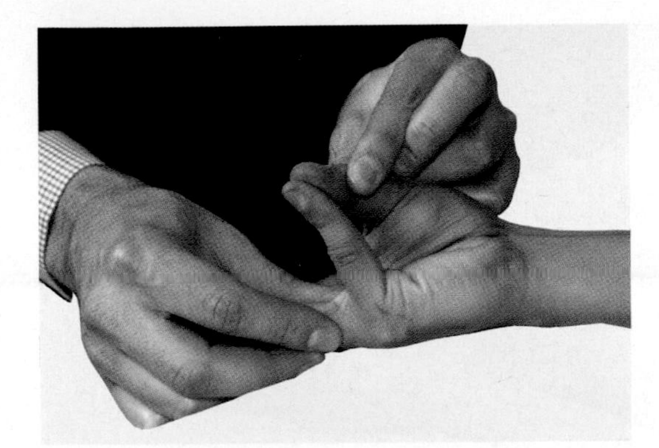

Figure 1–15 Opponens pollicis (C8, T1) assessment: Have the patient forcibly maintain contact between the volar pads of the distal thumb and fifth digit, while you try to pull the distal first metacarpal away from the fifth digit. Although thumb opposition is only innervated by the median nerve, a combination of thumb adduction (adductor pollicis, ulnar nerve) and thumb flexion (flexor pollicis brevis, deep head, ulnar nerve) may mimic thumb opposition even when there is complete median nerve palsy present.

substitution by the flexor pollicis longus occurs. Use your other hand to immobilize the first metacarpal to reduce substitution by the opponens pollicis. Because of its dual innervation, even with complete thenar motor branch palsies some thumb flexion should still occur. However, when compared with the normal hand, relative weakness is usually evident. Assess the *opponens pollicis* (C8, T1) by having the patient forcibly maintain contact between the volar pads of the distal thumb and fifth digit while you try to pull the distal first metacarpal away from the fifth digit (**Fig. 1–15**). Although the median nerve solely controls thumb opposition, a combination of thumb adduction (adductor pollicis, ulnar nerve) and thumb flexion (flexor pollicis brevis, deep head, ulnar nerve) may mimic thumb opposition when there is complete median nerve palsy present.

- **Examining the motor function of the thumb is not straightforward. The key principle is to compare the results with the normal hand, keeping in mind that even following complete loss of median nerve function, some movement of the thumb will still be present secondary to either true muscle action via radial and ulnar innervation, or from substitutions by adjacent muscles.**

The Terminal Group

The terminal group simply consists of the *first and second lumbricals* (C8, T1), which are innervated by the terminal radial and ulnar divisions of the median nerve, respectively. To examine the first lumbrical, stabilize the index finger in a hyper-extended position at the metacarpal-phalangeal joint and then provide resistance as the patient extends the finger at the proximal interphalangeal joint (**Fig. 1–16**).

- **The muscular origins and insertions of the lumbricals are quite variable. In fact, one or more may be absent. This variability and/or absence of the lumbricals is functionally acceptable because flexion at the**

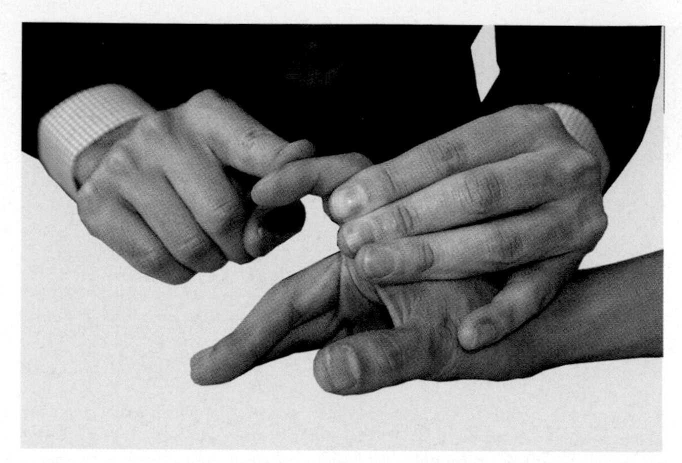

Figure 1–16 Lumbrical of second digit (C8, T1) assessment: Stabilize the patient's index finger in a hyper-extended position at the metacarpal-phalangeal joint and then provide resistance as the patient extends the finger at the proximal interphalangeal joint.

metacarpal-phalangeal joints, as well as extension at the proximal interphalangeal joints when the metacarpal-phalangeal joints are hyperextended (both movements performed by the lumbricals), are also partly performed by the palmar or dorsal interossei muscles. Therefore, whenever you test lumbrical strength, it is being assisted by the interossei.

♦ Sensory Innervation

Although the median nerve only provides sensory innervation to a relatively small portion of the upper extremity, it is probably the most important. Via three branches, the *palmar cutaneous nerve*, and the *radial and ulnar divisions of the median nerve* (via digital branches) in the palm, the median nerve carries cutaneous sensory information from the radial two thirds of the palm, and the volar surfaces of the first, second, third, and radial half of the fourth digits (**Fig. 1–17**). Dorsal fingertip sensation is also carried by the median nerve, including the dorsum of the ulnar half of the distal phalanx of the thumb, as well as the dorsum of the distal phalanges of the second, third, and radial half of the fourth digits.

The palmar cutaneous branch innervates the majority of the median nerve's palmar distribution, while that of the digits is through small branches of the median nerve's radial and ulnar divisions in the palm. Therefore, one should use the thenar eminence to assess the palmar cutaneous branch, and the distal portion of the second and third digits to assess the sensory fibers that pass through the carpal tunnel. In addition to sensory cutaneous innervation, the median nerve also carries sensory fibers for joint proprioception and muscle tension, especially from the elbow and wrist. Although many refer to the anterior

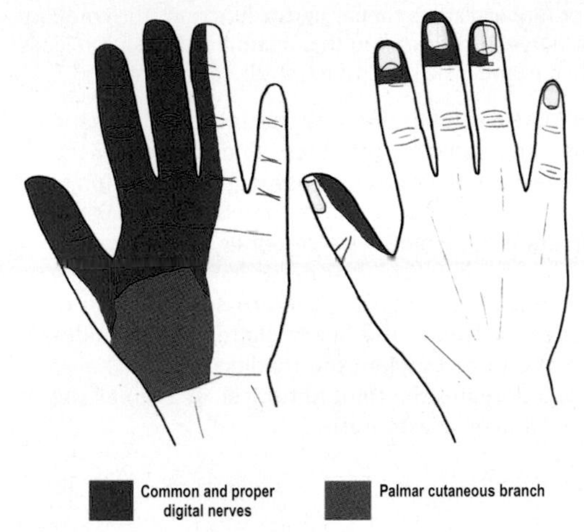

Figure 1–17 Sensory innervation of the median nerve. The median nerve carries cutaneous sensory information from the radial two thirds of the palm, and the volar surfaces of the first, second, third, and radial half of the fourth digit.

interosseous nerve as a "pure" motor nerve without cutaneous innervation, it does, in fact carry sensory fibers from the wrist joints and muscles.

- **The ulnar border of the median nerve's sensory innervation in the hand may vary, depending on its relationship, or dominance over, the adjacent ulnar nerve. For example, either the ulnar or the median nerve may receive sensory innervation from the complete volar fourth digit. Furthermore, the percentage of the palm's median innervated region carried by the palmar cutaneous branch versus branches of the radial and ulnar divisions of the median nerve is also variable.**

Martin–Gruber and Riche–Cannieu Anastomoses

Cross talk, or anastomoses, between the ulnar nerve and either the median nerve or its anterior interosseous branch may occur in the forearm. Many variations are possible, and knowing a few of the more common ones is clinically useful.

The *Martin–Gruber anastomosis* occurs in up to 15% of patients and involves the median innervated thenar muscles (opponens pollicis, abductor pollicis brevis, and flexor pollicis brevis). In this anomaly, instead of their usual pathway down the median nerve and out the thenar motor branch, nerve fibers destined for these three muscles run instead down the anterior interosseous branch, are transferred through the flexor digitorum profundus muscle to the ulnar nerve, and then enter the palm via the deep ulnar branch. Deep in the palm, these fibers are eventually transferred back to the thenar motor branch, where they innervate their respective muscles. This distal communication between the deep ulnar branch and the thenar motor branch in the palm is termed the *Riche–Cannieu anastomosis*, and is anatomically (not functionally) present in at least 50% of patients.

Therefore, when motor axons destined for the median nerve's thenar muscles cross over to the ulnar nerve via the Martin–Gruber anastomosis, low median nerve injuries in the wrist or forearm spare thenar motor function. The corollary is that damage to the ulnar nerve at the wrist in this anatomical situation leads to a much more severe deficit of intrinsic hand function than expected.

- **Another version of the Martin–Gruber anastomosis involves the hand intrinsic muscles usually innervated by the deep ulnar branch in the hand, including the lumbricals, first dorsal interosseous, adductor pollicis, and deep (ulnar) portion of the flexor pollicis brevis. For this variation, motor axons innervating these muscles accidentally pass down the median nerve and then pass back to the ulnar nerve halfway down the forearm via communications with the anterior interosseous branch of the median nerve, through or around the flexor digitorum profundus muscle. Yet another variation occurs when the median nerve's thenar motor branch aberrantly innervates the third lumbrical, or even all the lumbricals, via the Riche–Cannieu anastomosis**

♦ Clinical Findings and Syndromes

The Arm

Complete Palsy

Damage to the median nerve in the arm is usually secondary to trauma: lacerations, gunshots, or blunt contusions. Because of the median nerve's close proximity to the brachial artery, concomitant injury to this vessel may occur. Furthermore, in the proximal arm both the ulnar and radial nerves are in close proximity to the median nerve, and therefore, all three of these nerves can be simultaneously injured (*triad neuropathy*). The *Saturday night palsy*, which can occur from hanging the arm over the back of a chair and passing out (drunk), or the *honeymooners palsy*, which occurs when the arm is under the neck of someone sleeping for a length of time, can both cause a median nerve palsy. Although classically injuring the radial nerve, a crutch head can also damage the median nerve in the axilla.

A complete injury to the median nerve is debilitating. The forearm cannot pronate against gravity or resistance. The hand can only weakly flex at the wrist in an ulnar direction. The thumb cannot be opposed or abducted in a palmar direction. Lumbrical weakness in the index and long fingers is present. Numbness occurs on the volar surfaces of the first three and a half digits, and radial two thirds of the palm. Additionally, when a patient with a complete median palsy is asked to make a fist, the first digit barely flexes, the second digit partially flexes (secondary to substitution from nonmedian innervated muscles), the third digit flexes but is weak, while the fourth and fifth digits flex normally, which is called a *Benedictine sign* (or *orator's hand*) (**Fig. 1–18**). This sign of median nerve palsy is so named because of its similarity to the hand position during blessings, and is seen in many portraits of Jesus.

When examining a complete median nerve palsy, the following pitfalls must be considered. The brachioradialis (radial innervated), with the help of gravity, may pronate the forearm from full supination. You may be tricked into observing thumb opposition by the indirect actions of the flexor pollicis brevis (deep head) and the adductor pollicis (both ulnar innervated). Lastly, palmar abduction of the thumb may be falsely mimicked by the flexor pollicis brevis (deep

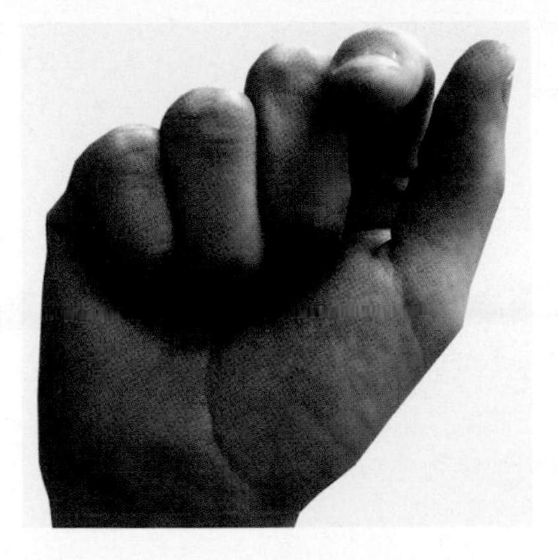

Figure 1–18 Benedictine sign. When a patient with a complete median palsy is asked to make a fist, the first digit barely flexes, the second digit partially flexes (secondary to substitution from non-median innervated muscles), the third digit flexes but is weak, while the fourth and fifth digits flex normally, creating what is known as the Benedictine sign.

head), or truly moved in radial abduction by the abductor pollicis longus (radial innervated).

Supracondylar Spur/Ligament of Struthers

Approximately 1% of people have a supracondylar spur on the medial side of the humerus about 5 cm proximal to the medial epicondyle. When this accessory condyle is present, it is thought that in most cases a ligament bridging it to the medial epicondyle is present. This ligament is called the *ligament of Struthers* after the anatomist who first described the supracondylar spur. When present, the median nerve usually passes underneath this ligament with either the brachial artery or its ulnar branch. This anatomically confined channel can cause median nerve entrapment in some patients (**Fig. 1–19**).

Clinically, this entrapment has been reported to cause insidious onset of forearm and hand weakness, with variable sensory loss in a median distribution. A deep aching pain is often present in the proximal forearm, which occasionally worsens with repetitive pronation/supination, or strength testing of the pronator teres or flexor carpi radialis. On examination, variable weakness, and even muscle wasting, may occur in any median nerve innervated muscle. Occasionally, the branches to the pronator teres arise proximal to the median nerve passing under the ligament of Struthers, and therefore, may be spared. Weakness of proximal forearm flexors, particularly the muscles innervated by the anterior interosseous nerve (ask the patient to make the okay sign), should be documented because this pattern of weakness frequently occurs in this entrapment (more below). A Tinel's sign in the distal, medial upper arm may be present. Of course, palpation or a radiograph confirming the presence of a supracondylar spur is also required to make this diagnosis.

Supracondylar Fractures

Supracondylar fractures usually occur in children, and may cause median nerve damage. This is especially true for displaced fractures. Delayed median palsies can also occur secondary to progressive callus formation. As mentioned for ligament of Struthers entrapment of the median nerve, supracondylar injuries often involve axons destined for the anterior interosseous nerve. This occurs for two reasons. First, the relatively fixed anterior interosseous nerve is placed on stretch when a fractured arm is displaced posteriorly. Second, the nerve fibers destined

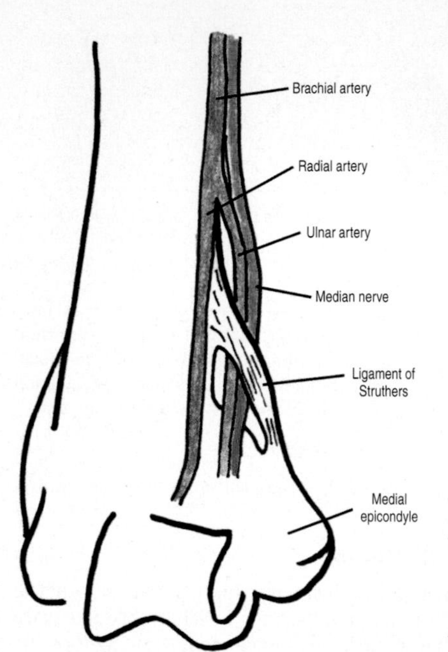

Figure 1–19 Ligament of Struthers. Approximately 1% of people have a supracondylar spur on the medial side of the humerus about 5 cm proximal to the medial epicondyle. When this accessory condyle is present, in most cases a ligament bridging this supracondylar spur to the medial epicondyle is present.

to the anterior interosseous nerve, along with the sensory fibers destined for the first two digits, are located posteriorly in the median nerve, and are prone to injury as it passes through the supracondylar region. When a patient has isolated anterior interosseous motor loss secondary to partial median nerve damage in the supracondylar region (not to the anterior interosseous branch), it is indicative of *pseudo-anterior interosseous neuropathy*. This more proximal damage also causes thumb and index finger numbness, which helps differentiate this injury from a true anterior interosseous neuropathy.

The Forearm

Musculotendinous Median Neuropathies

The bicipital aponeurosis, which crosses from lateral to medial over the antecubital fossa and serves to attach indirectly the biceps brachii tendon to the ulna, may irritate the median nerve. The pathogenesis of this is uncertain, but a thickened aponeurosis, hypertrophied brachialis (which lies under the median nerve and theoretically can push it superficially into the aponeurosis), or an anomalous muscle insertion of the pronator teres (which alters the local anatomic arrangements), may each predispose to this type of compression. Patients with bicipital aponeurosis entrapment have a similar presentation and exam to those with ligament of Struthers compression. They frequently report elbow pain radiating both proximally and distally. Occasionally, resisted forearm flexion in the supinated position for 30 seconds may precipitate symptoms. Of note, this compression is very rare.

The median nerve may be compressed or pinched where it passes between the two heads of the pronator teres (**Fig. 1–20**). This occurs most commonly in people who perform repetitive, forceful pronation of their forearm; it is called *pronator teres syndrome*. The only median-innervated muscle that cannot be affected by this syndrome is the pronator teres because branches from the median nerve destined for this muscle originate proximal to where the median nerve passes under this muscle. Pronator teres syndrome is characterized by an insidious onset of dull aching pain in the proximal forearm that is worsened by repetitive or forceful pronation. In fact, the most common finding is tenderness of the pronator teres to palpation. Median innervated hand sensation is often normal, and motor function may be difficult to ascertain because of pain. Nonetheless, weakness is occasionally seen during flexion of the second and third digits. A Tinel's sign can often be elicited at the antecubital fossa. In contradistinction to carpal tunnel syndrome, patients usually do not complain of nocturnal pain and/or numbness. The true incidence of this syndrome is unknown, and some authors suggest it should be separated into those with objective findings versus those without.

A fibrotic arch between the two heads of the flexor digitorum superficialis may also irritate the median nerve (**Fig. 1–20**). This ridge has been called the *sublimis arch*, and may compress the median nerve as it passes underneath. Clinical manifestation of this entrapment is quite similar to pronator teres syndrome, except that forceful flexion of the proximal interphalangeal joints of the second to fifth digits, which is mediated by contraction of the flexor digitorum superficialis muscle, may precipitate symptoms.

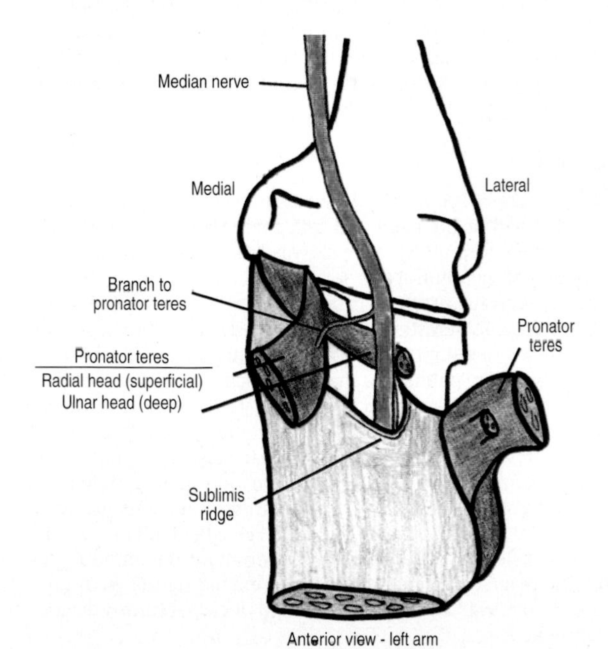

Figure 1–20 Pronator teres syndrome and sublimis arch. The median nerve may be compressed or pinched where it passes between the two heads of the pronator teres. A fibrotic arch may alternatively compress it when it passes under the two heads of the flexor digitorum superficialis.

Of note, with surgical treatment of median nerve entrapment at the elbow, all three possible compression points—bicipital aponeurosis, pronator teres, and sublimis arch—are each inspected and decompressed.

The Anterior Interosseous Nerve

An isolated palsy affecting the anterior interosseous nerve may occur secondary to trauma, fractures, Parsonage–Turner syndrome, anomalous muscles and/or tendons, or without known cause. Patients usually complain of weakness or clumsiness in grasping objects with their first two fingers (e.g., grasping the handle of a coffee cup). There are usually no complaints of pain, and because this nerve does not carry cutaneous sensation, no numbness occurs. Weakness of the flexor digitorum profundus (to the second and third digits), flexor pollicis longus, and pronator quadratus is present. Patients have a positive okay sign (**Fig. 1–11**). To confirm pure, anterior interosseous nerve palsy, all other median nerve innervated muscles, as well as sensation, must be normal. Partial anterior interosseous palsies are possible, as are partial median nerve palsies mimicking an anterior interosseus nerve deficit (pseudo-anterior interosseous neuropathy). Although anterior interosseous nerve palsy is a clinical diagnosis, magnetic resonance imaging (MRI) would show denervation of the three muscles innervated by this nerve.

- **Patients with rheumatoid arthritis can have spontaneous and painless rupture of the flexor digitorum profundus and flexor pollicis longus tendons, mimicking an anterior interosseous palsy. To exclude this possibility, have the patient open and relax the hand. If the tendons are intact, pressing your thumb firmly across the ventral aspect of the forearm about 2 to 3 inches proximal to the wrist should cause passive finger flexion.**

Carpal Tunnel Syndrome

The symptoms of carpal tunnel syndrome are well described: aching pain and paresthesias in the radial half of the palm and first three digits that wakes the patient up at night, and is relieved by "shaking it away." Of course, each patient's presentation is a variation of this central theme; perhaps it is only in the fingers, maybe they "don't shake it away," maybe it is only paresthesias or coldness, etc. On examination, hypesthesia, hyperesthesia, and/or diminished vibratory sense may be present in the first three digits. Remember, the majority of the median innervated palm region is via the palmar cutaneous branch, which does not pass through the carpal tunnel. Therefore, objective sensory testing on the thenar eminence is often normal; however, patients still commonly report pain and "abnormal" sensation in this area. In severe cases, thenar muscle wasting can be seen, as well as weakness in thumb opposition, flexion, and palmar abduction. Rarely, the thenar motor branch is selectively compressed. Other tests include a Tinel's sign at the wrist, and the Phalen's test and/or reverse Phalen's test. A positive Phalen's test is when flexing the affected wrist for about one minute precipitates symptoms. The reverse Phalen's test is when extending the wrist does the same. Dr. Phalen, of note, was a pioneer in the field of carpal tunnel diagnosis and surgical treatment.

The etiology of carpal tunnel syndrome is uncertain. Space-occupying lesions in this passage obviously may predispose one to this syndrome (e.g., ganglion cysts, anomalous lumbrical muscles, fractures, etc.). Certain systemic diseases are also associated with entrapment here, including diabetes, chronic dialysis treatment, rheumatoid arthritis, acromegaly, obesity, and hypothyroidism, to name a few. A genetic predisposition to carpal tunnel syndrome (familial carpal tunnel syndrome) has been reported; these patients are thought to have a small carpal tunnel and/or a thickened transverse carpal ligament.

As with other more common compression syndromes, the clinical situation may worsen or improve over time, rapidly or slowly. A simple grading system separating carpal tunnel syndrome into mild, moderate, and severe is useful for treatment decision-making and prognosis. *Mild* carpal tunnel syndrome includes complaints of numbness and tingling at night, and occasionally during the day. The most common area involved is the long finger followed by the palm. A significant portion of the day the patient's hand feels near normal. Pain is uncommon at this early stage. Two-point discrimination is usually okay, although vibration sense and light touch may actually be heightened in the affected fingers. No weakness or atrophy is present. In *moderate* carpal tunnel syndrome, the symptoms are more pervasive throughout the day. Sensory testing now reveals hypesthesia to light touch and vibration. Two-point discrimination may be abnormal. A Tinel's sign is now present at the wrist, and a positive Phalen's test may occur. Muscle weakness is still not present. In *severe* carpal tunnel syndrome, the patient's symptoms are constant, weakness and atrophy may occur, and a Tinel's sign at this point may even be absent secondary to extensive nerve damage. To reiterate, mild carpal tunnel syndrome is a diagnosis of medical history, with physical findings not usually present; moderate cases have sensory abnormalities and likely a Tinel's sign; and severe cases have constant sensory symptoms and perhaps motor weakness.

2

The Diagnostic Anatomy of the Ulnar Nerve

The ulnar nerve innervates most of the hand intrinsic muscles, and therefore is the nerve that is predominantly responsible for controlling fine, coordinated hand movements. Otherwise, the ulnar nerve innervates no muscles in the upper arm, and only two in the forearm. It does not travel in the midline like the median nerve, but instead takes a direct, yet hidden, route from the axilla down to the hypothenar eminence. From proximal to distal, the ulnar nerve hides in the medial head of the triceps, passes along the backside of the elbow, runs down the forearm under the flexor carpi ulnaris, and enters finally into Guyon's tunnel at the wrist. Commensurate with its surreptitious approach to the deep palmar area, a severe ulnar deficit can manifest itself as a claw hand. The most common location of ulnar nerve entrapment is not at the wrist, like for the median nerve, but instead behind the elbow, where the ulnar nerve is superficial and vulnerable to dynamic compression.

♦ Anatomical Course

The Arm

The brachial plexus cords are named based on their relationship to the axillary artery under the pectoralis minor, and because the ulnar nerve is a continuation of the medial cord, it naturally begins (and remains) medial to the axillary artery. After its contribution to the median nerve, the medial cord continues distally as the ulnar nerve. The ulnar nerve comprises predominantly fibers from the C8 and T1 spinal nerves. However, C7 input may also be present (see below).

The transformation of the medial and lateral cords into their terminal branches is M-shaped, and lies over the anterior aspect of the axillary artery. The lateral leg of the letter M is the musculocutaneous nerve; the medial leg is the ulnar nerve. The center, V-shaped, convergence consists of components of the lateral and medial cords merging to become the median nerve (**Fig. 2–1**).

Before the medial cord becomes the ulnar nerve, it yields two important sensory branches, the *medial brachial cutaneous* and *medial antebrachial cutaneous* nerves, which innervate the medial half of the arm and forearm, respectively (**Fig. 2–2**). Despite being branches from the medial cord, for simplicity's sake, these nerves will be considered part of the ulnar nerve's sensory territory. If one considers these two nerves as "very proximal" branches of the ulnar nerve, then

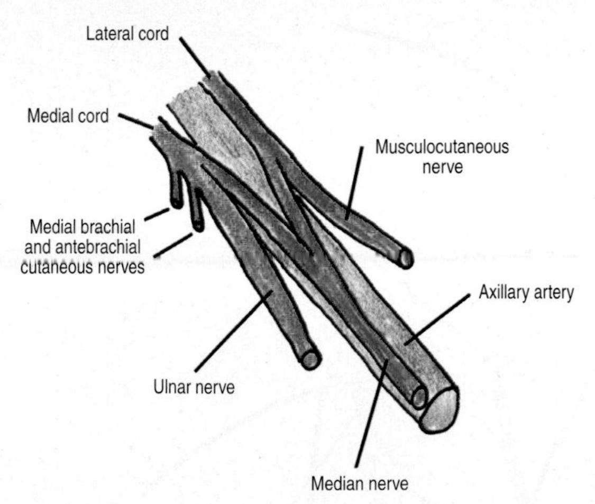

Figure 2–1 Origin of the ulnar nerve in the axilla. The transformation of the medial and lateral cords into their terminal branches is M-shaped, and lies over the anterior aspect of the axillary artery. The lateral leg of the letter M is the musculocutaneous nerve; the medial leg is the ulnar nerve. The center, V-shaped convergence consists of contributions from the lateral and medial cords merging to become the median nerve.

one can simply say that the ulnar nerve's sensory territory is the medial half of the whole upper limb, including the hand.

The medial brachial cutaneous nerve pierces the superficial fascia of the arm near the axilla and then runs in the subcutaneous space innervating the medial surface of the arm. The distal portion of this nerve may reach an area posterior to the medial epicondyle, and in this region be inadvertently transected during ulnar nerve decompressions.

The medial antebrachial cutaneous nerve branches into an anterior and posterior branch just proximal, and anterior, to the medial epicondyle. Near this area of bifurcation, components of this nerve pierce the superficial fascia of the arm and enter the subcutaneous space. The anterior division runs along the anteromedial forearm, while the posterior branch runs along the posteromedial aspect of the forearm. The posterior branch *often* crosses the field of operative exposure for decompression of the ulnar nerve, while the anterior branch can be harmed when the median nerve is exposed in the antecubital fossa.

Down the upper half of the arm, the ulnar nerve runs along the brachial artery's medial aspect, opposite the median nerve, which runs on the brachial artery's lateral side (**Fig. 2–3**). Proximally, the ulnar nerve lies on the anterior border of the intermuscular septum, a thick fascial plane that separates the flexor and extensor compartments of the arm. At about the coracobrachialis muscle's insertion into the humerus, which occurs halfway down the arm, the ulnar nerve pierces this intermuscular septum. The superior ulnar collateral artery, a branch from the brachial artery, runs with the ulnar nerve through this septum. Once piercing the intermuscular septum, the ulnar nerve becomes enveloped within the anteromedial aspect of the medial head of the triceps, inside of which it continues down the arm. In approximately 50% of persons, an extension of the intermuscular septum forms an arch, or arcade, that attaches to the medial head of the triceps. This structure is a few centimeters in length and is termed the

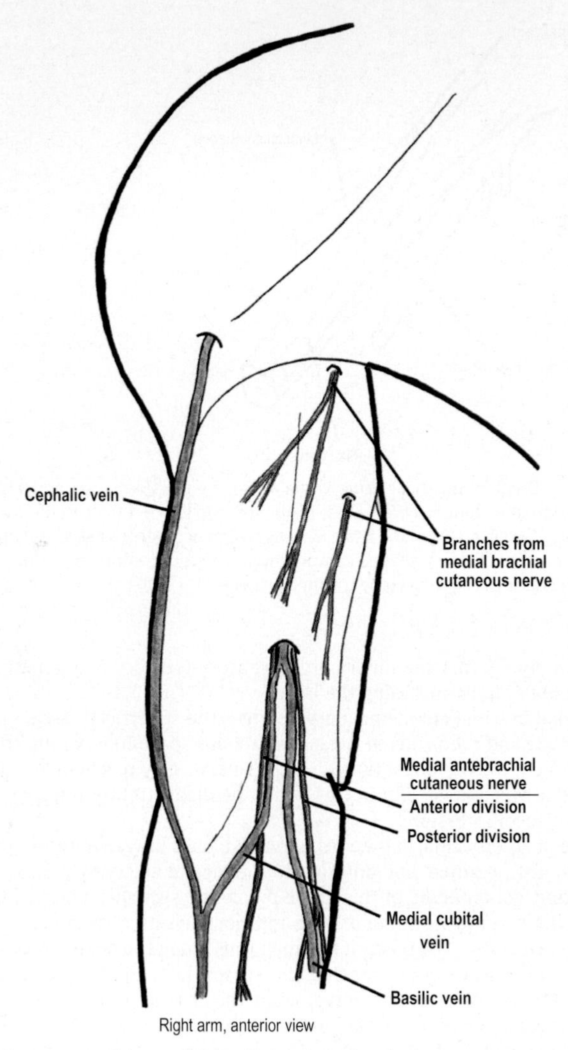

Figure 2–2 Course of the medial brachial and antebrachial cutaneous nerves. Before the medial cord becomes the ulnar nerve, it yields two important sensory branches, the medial brachial cutaneous and medial antebrachial cutaneous nerves, which innervate the medial half of the arm and forearm, respectively.

arcade of Struthers, and is located about two thirds of the way down the arm. The ulnar nerve, which is deep and enveloped in the medial triceps head, runs under this arcade, when present. The arcade of Struthers should not be confused with the ligament of Struthers, which bridges an anomalous supracondylar ridge on the distal humeral shaft to the medial humeral epicondyle (see median nerve chapter). As the medial head of the triceps narrows into its distal tendon, the

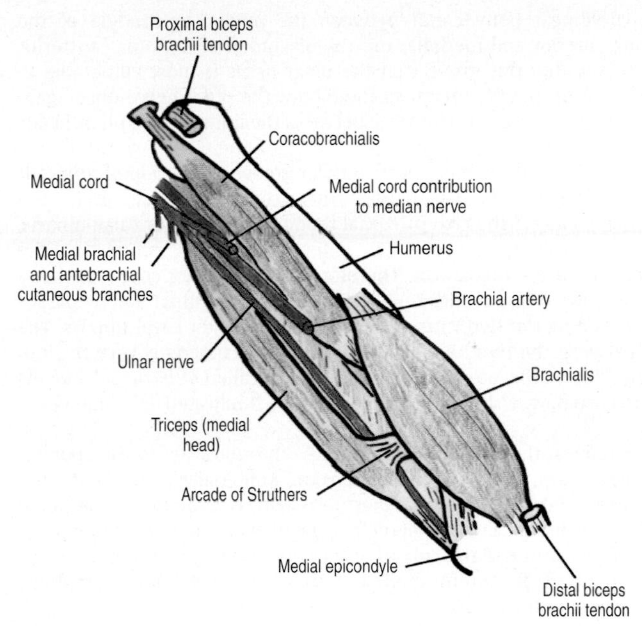

Figure 2–3 The course of the ulnar nerve in the arm. In the proximal arm, the ulnar nerve lies on the anterior border of the intermuscular septum. Once piercing the intermuscular septum, the ulnar nerve becomes enveloped within the anteromedial aspect of the medial head of the triceps, inside of which it continues down the arm.

ulnar nerve emerges from its passage within this muscle and enters the posteromedial elbow region. The inferior ulnar artery, which also arises from the brachial artery, joins the ulnar nerve at this level. Branches of the inferior ulnar artery adhere to, and pass with, the ulnar nerve through the elbow region.

The mobility of the ulnar nerve changes as it passes down the medial arm. When anterior to the intermuscular septum in the upper half of the arm the ulnar nerve is mobile. However, it subsequently becomes immobilized in the lower half of the arm by being imbedded in the triceps muscle, and under the arcade of Struthers, when present. The ulnar nerve becomes once again mobile just proximal to the postcondylar groove of the elbow.

- **In many individuals, there is a C7 contribution to the ulnar nerve, which originates from the lateral cord. This neural communication within the brachial plexus has been labeled *the lateral root of the ulnar nerve*. In a minority of people the antebrachial cutaneous nerve, or even the more proximal medial brachial cutaneous nerve, can originate directly from the ulnar nerve, providing another reason for these sensory branches to be categorized with the ulnar nerve.**

The Elbow

After emerging from the medial head of the triceps in the lower arm, the ulnar nerve runs subcutaneously and enters the postcondylar groove. This groove is a curvilinear bony canal between the medial epicondyle of the humerus (lying anterior and medial), and the olecranon of the ulna (posterior and lateral). It is within this grove that the ulnar nerve is most vulnerable to external trauma. After passing distal to the elbow, the ulnar nerve once again dives below a protective muscle, this time between the humeral and ulnar heads of the flexor carpi ulnaris.

This region, just beyond the bony postcondylar groove, is the *cubital tunnel*. It has two segments (**Fig. 2–4**): The first is where the nerve passes under the aponeurosis that connects the two proximal tendons of the flexor carpi ulnaris. Although variable, this aponeurosis can extend proximally, connecting the medial epicondyle to the olecranon. Therefore, it may in fact cover the bony postcondylar groove. The second segment is where the ulnar nerve passes between, and deep to, the two muscular heads of the flexor carpi ulnaris. The aponeurosis between the two heads of the flexor carpi ulnaris is very thick in approximately 75% of the population, and is then called *Osborne's band*. As will be discussed below, Osborne's band has been implicated in ulnar nerve compression.

Dynamic anatomy at the elbow is important. As the elbow flexes, the aponeurosis of the flexor carpi ulnaris is under tension, potentially compressing the ulnar nerve underneath (**Fig. 2–5**). Furthermore, with contraction of the flexor carpi ulnaris muscle itself, the ulnar nerve may be further compressed under the second, more distal, portion of the cubital tunnel. This is partly why simultaneous elbow flexion and wrist flexion in an ulnar direction can precipitate symptoms of ulnar entrapment at the elbow.

- **The amount of aponeurosis covering the postcondylar groove, as well as the space between the two heads of the flexor carpi ulnaris, is variable. In fact, some patients may not have this covering at all, allowing the ulnar nerve to slip, or "snap" over the medial epicondyle during forearm flexion.**

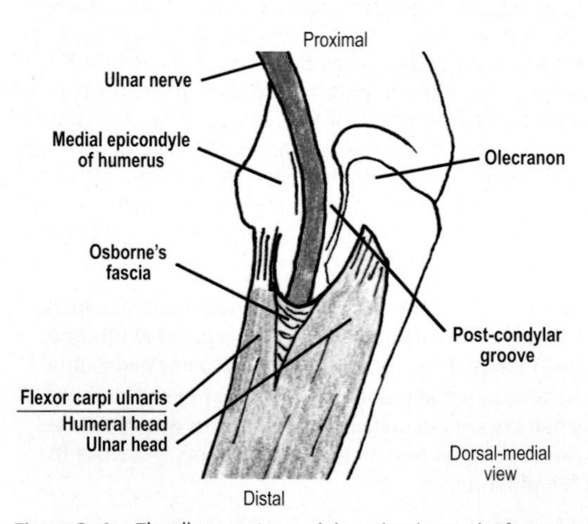

Figure 2–4 The elbow region and the cubital tunnel. After exiting the postcondylar groove, the ulnar nerve travels through the cubital tunnel. In approximately 75% of the population, the superficial aponeurosis between the two heads of the flexor carpi ulnaris is very thick, and is called Osborne's band or fascia.

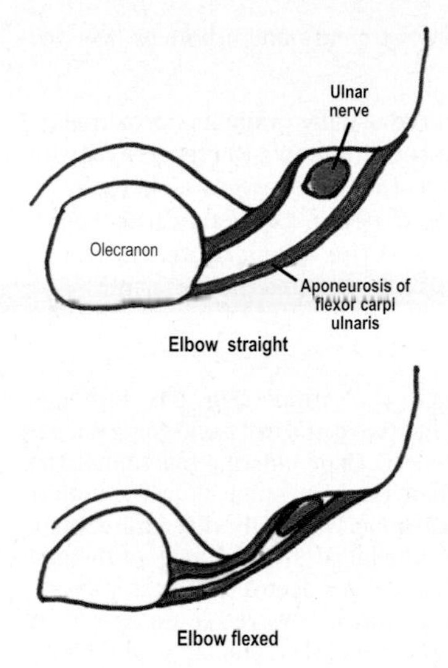

Figure 2–5 As the forearm flexes at the elbow, the area of the cubital tunnel decreases. Furthermore, with contraction of the flexor carpi ulnaris, the submuscular portion of the cubital tunnel also constricts (not shown). This is why simultaneous forearm flexion and wrist flexion in an ulnar direction can precipitate symptoms of ulnar entrapment at the elbow.

The anconeus epitrochlearis muscle is present in approximately 10% of the population. This muscle spans from the medial epicondyle to the olecranon, and is a potential cause of ulnar nerve irritation.

The Forearm

After passing deep to the two proximal heads of the flexor carpi ulnaris, the ulnar nerve continues down the forearm between this muscle superficially and the flexor digitorum profundus below. The ulnar nerve usually provides only one major branch to the flexor digitorum profundus, which arises after the branches destined for the flexor carpi ulnaris have already exited. The ulnar nerve passes in a direct trajectory from the medial epicondyle to the pisiform bone in the wrist. In the distal third of the forearm, the ulnar nerve emerges from between the flexor carpi ulnaris and flexor digitorum profundus, where these two muscles become tendinous. At this point, the ulnar nerve is not covered by muscle and lies between the flexor carpi ulnaris tendon medially, and the flexor digitorum superficialis tendon laterally. The ulnar artery, a branch from the brachial artery in the antecubital fossa, gradually makes its way medially to pair up with the ulnar nerve proximal to the wrist. Once together, these two structures enter the hand, with the artery lateral to the nerve.

Two sensory branches originate from the ulnar nerve in the distal half of the forearm. The first is the *dorsal ulnar cutaneous nerve*, which arises approximately 5 to 10 cm proximal to the wrist crease off the dorsomedial aspect of the ulnar nerve. This branch travels to the dorsum of the distal forearm between the ulna and the tendon of the flexor carpi ulnaris. Once on the dorsal surface, it pierces the antebrachial fascia and becomes subcutaneous a few centimeters proximal to the wrist. The second sensory branch from the ulnar nerve is the *palmar ulnar cutaneous nerve*, which is a mirror image of the palmar cutaneous branch of the median nerve. The palmar ulnar cutaneous nerve branches from the ulnar nerve approximately 5 to 10 cm proximal to the wrist from its volar-lateral surface and runs adherent to the ulnar nerve for a few centimeters. This branch enters the subcutaneous space proximal to the distal wrist crease and arborizes over the hypothenar eminence.

♦ **Although the dorsal ulnar cutaneous nerve usually originates proximal to the palmar ulnar cutaneous nerve, in certain people the reverse may be true. Alternatively, the dorsal ulnar cutaneous nerve may actually branch from the superficial sensory radial nerve. Communication, or "cross talk," between the ulnar nerve and the anterior interosseous nerve via the Martin–Gruber anastomosis may occur in the forearm.**

The Wrist/Hand

The ulnar nerve and artery enter the hand via Guyon's tunnel (**Fig. 2–6**). Although Guyon's tunnel has one proximal entrance, it has two distal exits, one going deeper into the hand, and the other remaining superficial. Upon entering this tunnel, the following structures are encountered. First, there is a large bump along the middle one half of the medial tunnel wall: the pisiform bone. Next at the distal third, there is another bump, but now on the lateral side: the hook of the hamate. At the end of the tunnel, there is a fork. The lateral pathway dives deep and almost immediately takes a sharp lateral bend. The medial pathway, however, continues in the same plane as the more proximal tunnel. In reviewing the boundaries of Guyon's tunnel, one needs to consider its proximal and distal segments separately. Please note that in the following discussion, medial refers to the hypothenar margin of the hand and lateral refers to the thenar aspect of the hand.

In the proximal half of Guyon's tunnel, the floor comprises the transverse carpal ligament and the roof the more superficial palmar carpal ligament (**Fig. 2–7**). The small palmaris brevis muscle also runs in the proximal roof of Guyon's tunnel. By passing deeper on the lateral margin of Guyon's tunnel, the superficial palmar carpal ligament briefly fuses with the transverse carpal ligament, thereby actually forming the lateral wall of Guyon's tunnel. However, the superficial palmar carpal ligament is the lateral wall for only the proximal portion of the tunnel. The flexor carpi ulnaris tendon and the more distal pisiform bone (first bump in the wall described earlier) form the proximal, medial wall of the tunnel.

For the distal half of the tunnel, the lateral wall is formed by the hook of the hamate (second bump in the wall described previously), and the shorter medial wall by the pisiform bone. The distal floor is formed initially by the

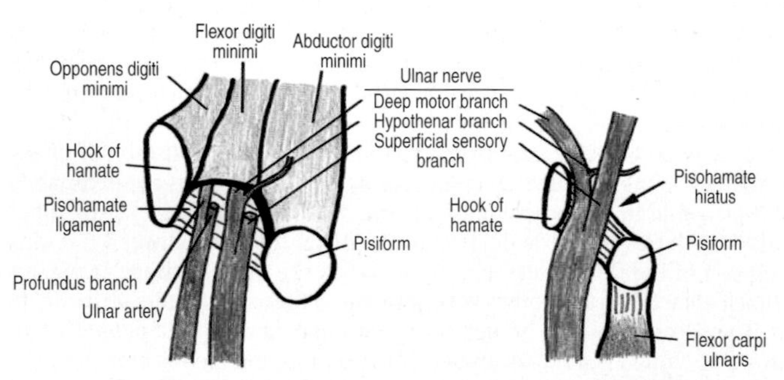

Figure 2–6 The ulnar nerve at the wrist. The ulnar nerve and artery enter the hand via Guyon's tunnel. Although Guyon's tunnel has one proximal entrance, it has two distal exits, one going deeper into the hand, and the other remaining superficial.

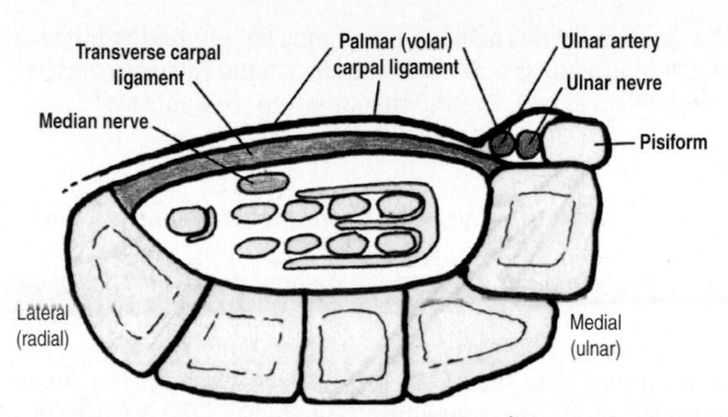

Figure 2–7 Proximal cross section of Guyon's tunnel. In the proximal half of Guyon's tunnel, the floor comprises the transverse carpal ligament and the roof the more superficial palmar carpal ligament. By passing deeper on the lateral margin of Guyon's tunnel, the superficial palmar carpal ligament fuses with the transverse carpal ligament, thereby also forming the lateral wall of Guyon's tunnel.

pisohamate ligament, then by the pisometacarpal ligament. The ulnar nerve passes superficial to both of these ligaments. The distal roof of Guyon's tunnel continues to be formed by the palmar carpal ligament. However, a muscular arch of the hypothenar muscle mass, from the pisiform to the hook of the hamate, forms the roof of the deeper, distal branch tunnel. This muscular arch is mainly made up of the flexor digiti minimi. Entrance to this deeper branch tunnel has been termed the *pisohamate hiatus*.

The ulnar nerve bifurcates into a deep motor branch and a superficial sensory branch in the distal portion of Guyon's tunnel. As their names imply, the superficial branch courses through the medial, more superficial tunnel with the main portion of the ulnar artery, while the deep branch goes down, with a profunda or deep branch of the ulnar artery, under the arch created by the flexor digiti minimi. This deep branch often pierces the opponens digiti muscle, but gives off a small side branch that innervates the hypothenar muscles just prior to it entering this deep passage. Once passing through Guyon's tunnel into the hand, the deep motor branch curves lateral toward the midline of the hand and thenar eminence, remaining deep to the flexor tendons of the fingers. The superficial branch splits into digital nerves to the fourth and fifth digits.

♦ **Occasionally, there may be early branching of the ulnar nerve with an anomalous course. For example, the ulnar nerve may branch proximal to the pisiform bone, with the superficial sensory branch communicating some, or all, of its sensory fibers to the palmar ulnar cutaneous nerve. A second variation occurs when the deep motor branch bifurcates prior to entering the pisohamate hiatus, with one branch entering the carpal tunnel lateral to the hook of the hamate, only to rejoin the deep branch in the palm.**

♦ Motor Innervation and Testing

As mentioned earlier, the ulnar nerve innervates no muscles in the upper arm, but is predominantly responsible for fine, coordinated hand and finger movements

(**Fig. 2–8**). The muscles innervated by the ulnar nerve may be grouped as follows: forearm (two muscles), hypothenar group (four muscles), hand intrinsic muscles or *intrinsics* (three *groups* of muscles), and the thenar group (two muscles).

The Forearm Group

The first muscle innervated by the ulnar nerve is the *flexor carpi ulnaris* (C7-T1). Branches to this muscle originate in the cubital tunnel, or just distal to it. Testing this muscle is a two-step process. First, while the patient abducts the ipsilateral fifth digit, observe and palpate the flexor carpi ulnaris' tendon just proximal to the wrist (**Fig. 2–9**). The flexor carpi ulnaris contracts to stabilize the pisiform so that the abductor digiti minimi may function. Next, have the patient flex his or her wrist against resistance in an ulnar direction (**Fig. 2–10**), which is the primary action of this muscle.

The second muscle innervated by the ulnar nerve in the forearm is the *flexor digitorum profundus* (C8, T1) to the fourth and fifth digits. Branches to this muscle originate when the ulnar nerve is between the flexor digitorum profundus and the flexor carpi ulnaris in the proximal forearm. This muscle is tested in the same fashion as for its median innervated half, except one uses the fifth digit: Immobilize the proximal interphalangeal joint while the patient flexes the distal interphalangeal joint (**Fig. 2–11**).

- **In 5% of patients, branches to the flexor carpi ulnaris originate proximal to the elbow. Although the median nerve's anterior interosseous branch may occasionally control distal interphalangeal joint flexion of the ring finger (in addition to the index and long fingers), the ulnar nerve always controls this movement in the fifth digit.**

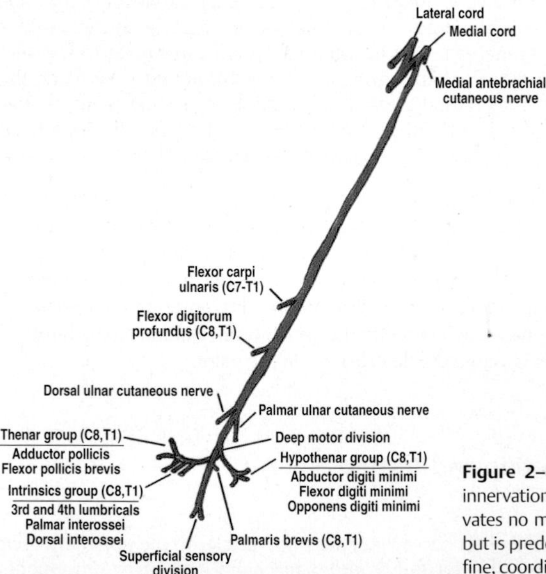

Figure 2–8 Ulnar nerve motor innervation. The ulnar nerve innervates no muscles in the upper arm, but is predominantly responsible for fine, coordinated finger movements.

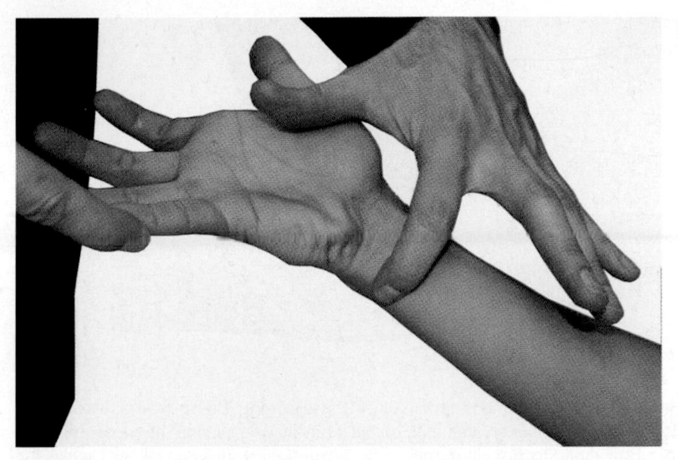

Figure 2–9 Flexor carpi ulnaris (C7–T1) assessment, stabilizing the pisiform: While the patient abducts the ipsilateral fifth digit, observe and palpate the flexor carpi ulnaris' tendon just proximal to the wrist. The flexor carpi ulnaris contracts to stabilize the pisiform so that the abductor digiti minimi may function.

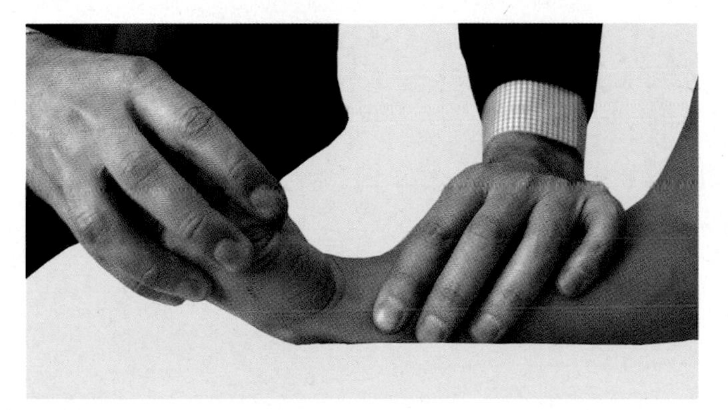

Figure 2–10 Flexor carpi ulnaris (C7-T1) assessment, wrist flexion: Have the patient flex his or her wrist against resistance in an ulnar direction, which is the primary action of this muscle.

The Hypothenar Group

As described, the ulnar nerve bifurcates into two divisions within Guyon's tunnel: the superficial sensory and deep motor. The superficial sensory division innervates only one, often-forgotten muscle, the *palmaris brevis* (C8, T1). The small branch that innervates this muscle usually originates from the sensory division as it leaves the distal end of Guyon's tunnel. The palmaris brevis is located in the roof of Guyon's tunnel, and when contracted, corrugates the hypothenar skin. This deepens the hollow of the hand, possibly aiding in grasp. To test this muscle, have the patient forcibly abduct the fifth digit and ask them to "contract" the hypothenar eminence. Skin corrugation should occur (**Fig. 2–12**).

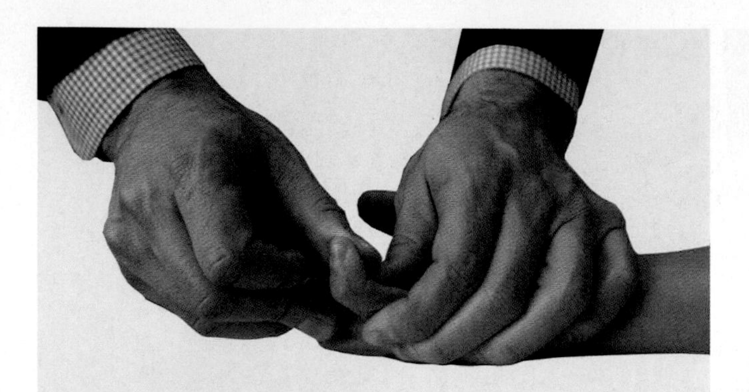

Figure 2–11 Flexor digitorum profundus (C8, T1) assessment: This muscle is tested in the same fashion as its median innervated half, except to evaluate the ulnar nerve contribution one uses the fifth digit. To test, immobilize the proximal interphalangeal joint while the patient flexes the distal interphalangeal joint against resistance.

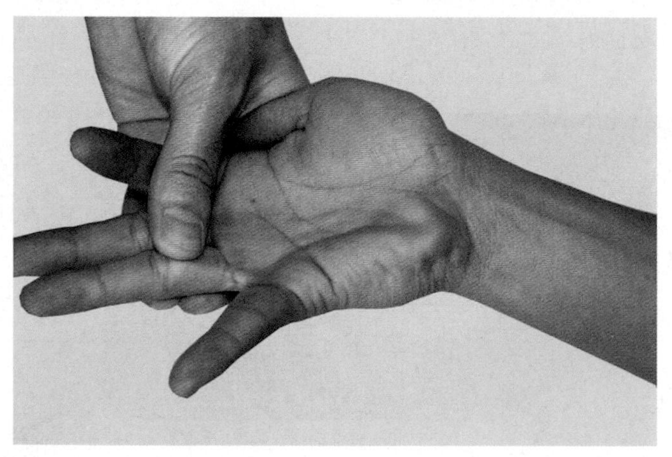

Figure 2–12 Palmaris brevis (C8, T1) assessment: Test this muscle by having the patient forcibly abduct the fifth digit and then instructing them to "contract" the hypothenar eminence simultaneously. Skin corrugation should occur.

The deep motor division gives a small motor branch to the hypothenar eminence just before diving into the pisohamate hiatus. This branch innervates the three muscles of the hypothenar eminence: the abductor digiti minimi, flexor digiti minimi, and the opponens digiti minimi. The *abductor digiti minimi* (C8, T1) is tested when the patient abducts the fifth digit against resistance (**Fig. 2–13**). One should keep in mind that this muscle is delicate, with even normal strength being easily overcome. The *flexor digiti minimi* (C8, T1) may be assessed by immobilizing the interphalangeal joints of the fifth digit, and instructing the patient to flex the metacarpal-phalangeal joint against resistance (**Fig. 2–14**). One cannot isolate this muscle's function, however, because flexion of the fifth digit's metacarpal-phalangeal joint is performed not only by the flexor digiti

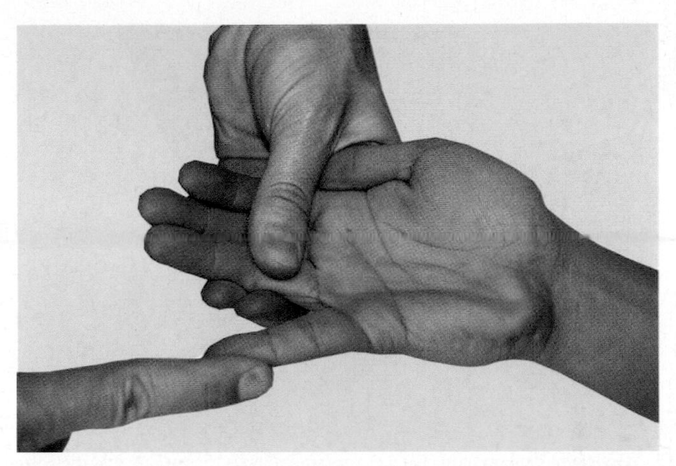

Figure 2–13 Abductor digiti minimi (C8, T1) assessment: This muscle is tested when the patient abducts the fifth digit against resistance. One should keep in mind that this muscle is delicate, the patient's resistance is easily overcome even with normal strength.

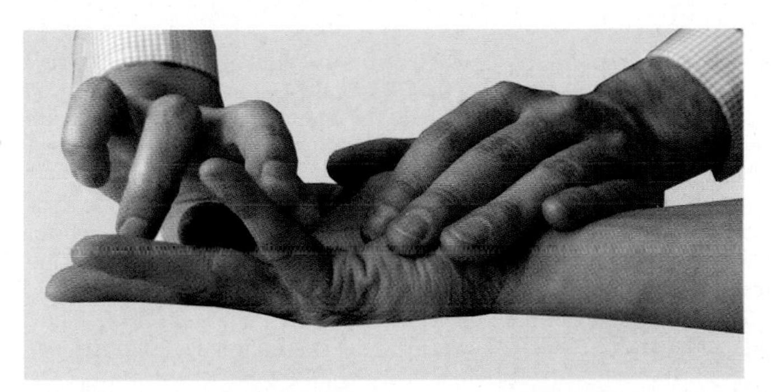

Figure 2–14 Flexor digiti minimi (C8, T1) assessment: This muscle is tested by immobilizing the interphalangeal joints of the fifth digit and having the patient flex the metacarpal-phalangeal (knuckle) joint against resistance. One cannot isolate this muscle's function, however, because flexion of the fifth digit's metacarpal-phalangeal joint is performed by not only the flexor digiti minimi, but also by the fourth lumbrical and the interossei.

minimi, but also by the fourth lumbrical, and the interossei. Next, test the *opponens digiti minimi* (C8, T1) by having the patient hold the volar pads of the distal thumb and fifth digit together. While the patient maintains this position, try to force the distal fifth metacarpal away from the thumb (**Fig. 2–15**). Hypothenar wasting may be evident with chronic denervation of these muscles.

The Hand Intrinsic Muscles

The small and deeply situated hand intrinsic muscles can be placed into three groups: the lumbricals, the palmar interossei, and the dorsal interossei. The lumbricals help flex the metacarpal-phalangeal joints and extend the proximal interphalangeal joints when the metacarpal-phalangeal joints are immobilized

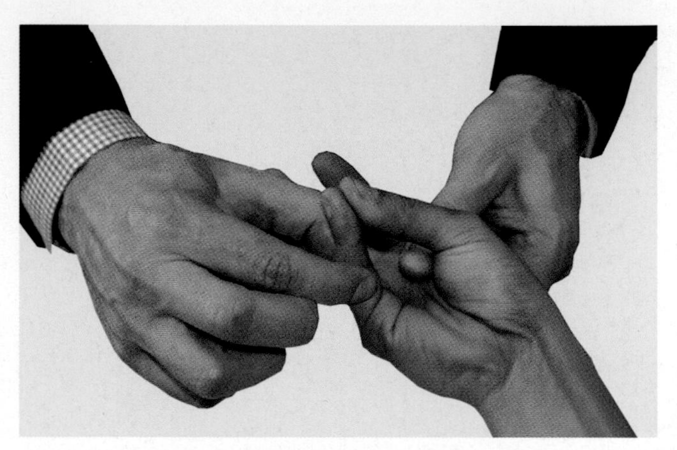

Figure 2–15 Opponens digiti minimi (C8, T1) assessment: Have the patient hold the volar pads of the distal thumb and fifth digit together. While the patient maintains this position, try to force the proximal digit and distal fifth metacarpal away from the thumb.

in a hyperextended position. The dorsal interossei abduct or spread the fingers. The palmar interossei adduct or close the fingers; they also assist the lumbricals in flexing the metacarpal-phalangeal joints. The deep branch of the ulnar nerve innervates the third and fourth lumbricals (to the fourth and fifth digits), as well as all of the palmar and dorsal interossei muscles.

To test the *third and fourth lumbricals* (C8, T1), immobilize the metacarpal-phalangeal joints of these two fingers in hyperextension and then test extension of the proximal interphalangeal joints against resistance (**Fig. 2–16**). A simple way to test the interossei is to concentrate on the index finger. On a flat surface have the patient both abduct (*first dorsal interosseus* [C8, T1], **Fig. 2–17**) or adduct (*second palmar interosseous* [C8, T1], **Fig. 2–18**) the index finger against resistance.

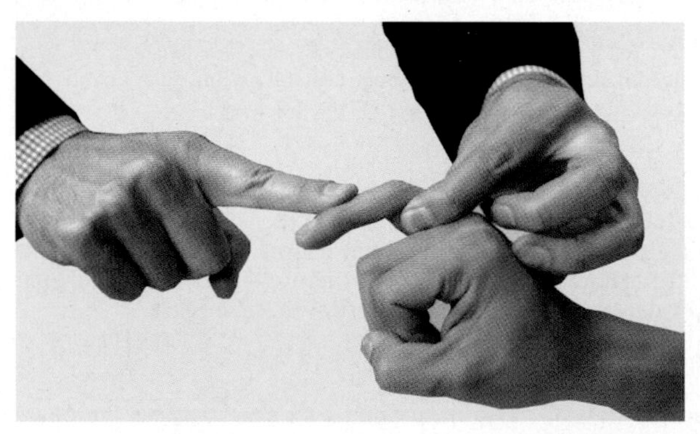

Figure 2–16 Third and fourth lumbrical (C8, T1) assessment: Immobilize the metacarpal-phalangeal joints of these two fingers in hyperextension and then test extension of the proximal interphalangeal joints against resistance.

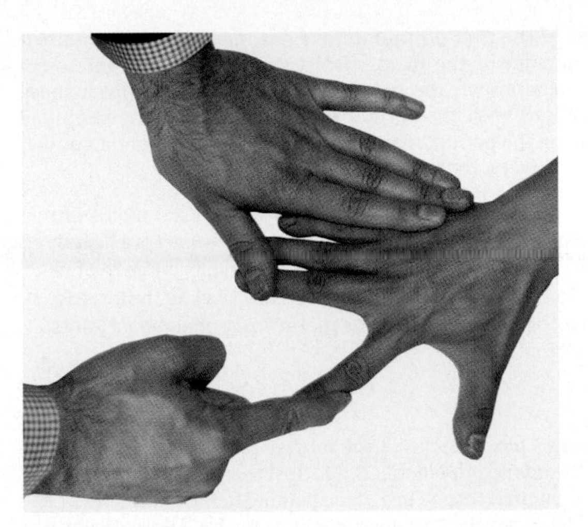

Figure 2–17 First dorsal interosseous (C8, T1) assessment: On a flat surface, the patient abducts his or her index finger against resistance. Contraction or atrophy of the first dorsal interosseous muscle can be observed and palpated on the dorsum of the hand.

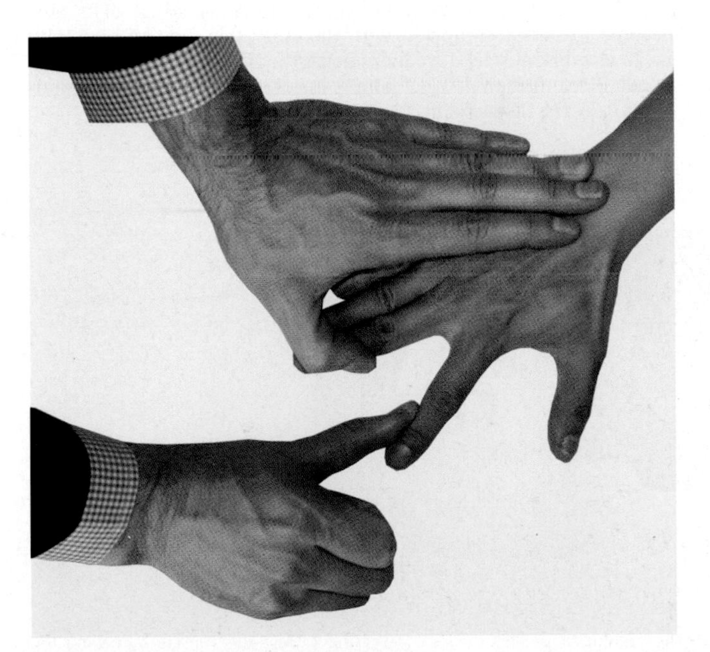

Figure 2–18 Second palmar interosseous (C8, T1) assessment: On a flat surface, the patient adducts the index finger against resistance. Alternatively, the patient can be instructed to keep the extended fingers together as the you attempt to pass a digit between them (not shown).

Contraction or atrophy of the first dorsal interosseous muscle can be observed and palpated on the dorsum of the hand. Also secondary to dorsal interossei wasting, the extensor tendons on the dorsum of the hand may appear more prominent when compared with the normal hand. The palmar interossei may also be assessed by having the patient maintain extended fingers together as you attempt to pass a digit between them.

- **The long finger flexors (flexor digitorum superficialis and flexor digitorum profundus) can substitute for digit adduction when the fingers are flexed. The finger extensors, in corollary, can help abduct the digits when the fingers are extended. To eliminate these substitutions and isolate the interossei, the fingers should be in extension at the metacarpal-phalangeal joints when assessed.**

The Thenar Group

The ulnar nerve innervates two muscles of the median nerve-dominated thenar eminence. The first is the *adductor pollicis* (C8, T1). Test this muscle by having the patient adduct the straightened thumb in a plane parallel to the palm (**Fig. 2–19**). Try to separate the thumb from the lateral border of the palm. Alternatively, you may place your index finger between his or her thumb and lateral palm, applying resistance as the thumb is adducted. Because of its large size, atrophy of this muscle alone may cause thenar wasting. The second muscle is the deep head of the *flexor pollicis brevis* (C8, T1), with its superficial head being innervated by the median nerve. Although not a very useful muscle to test because of its dual innervation, some weakness compared with the other side may be seen with ulnar lesions. To test this muscle, the patient flexes the thumb's metacarpal-phalangeal joint, while the interphalangeal joint is maintained in extension to minimize substitution by the flexor pollicis longus muscle (**Fig. 2–20**).

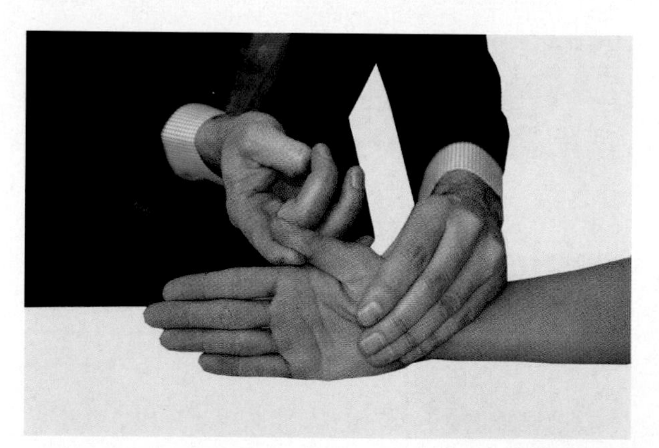

Figure 2–19 Adductor pollicis (C8, T1) assessment: Test this muscle by having the patient adduct a straightened thumb in the plane parallel to the palm. Try to separate the thumb from the lateral border of the palm. Alternatively, you may place your index finger between his or her thumb and lateral palm, applying resistance as the thumb is adducted (shown).

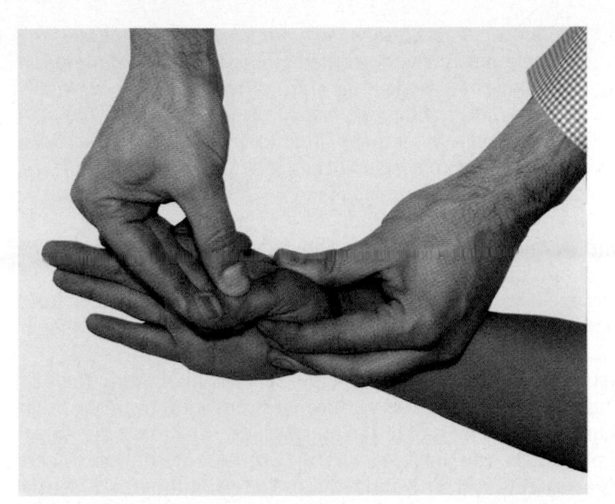

Figure 2–20 Flexor pollicis brevis (C8, T1) assessment: Although not a very useful muscle to test because of its dual innervation (median and ulnar nerves), some weakness compared with the other side may be seen with ulnar lesions. To test this muscle, the patient flexes the thumb's metacarpal-phalangeal joint, while the interphalangeal joint is maintained in extension to minimize substitution by the flexor pollicis longus muscle.

Martin–Gruber and Riche–Cannieu Anastomoses

As mentioned in the median nerve chapter, the median and ulnar nerves may communicate with each other in the forearm between the anterior interosseus nerve and the ulnar nerve (Martin–Gruber anastomosis). A second communication may occur in the deep palm between the thenar motor branch of the median nerve and the deep motor division of the ulnar nerve (Riche–Cannieu anastomosis). It is through these two potential routes of communication that minor or major shifts in motor innervation of the hand may occur.

The Riche–Cannieu anastomosis, although anatomically present in the majority of patients, does not always communicate axons that shift innervation between median and ulnar nerves. However, when transfer does occur, this connection most commonly either returns thenar innervation that was transferred to the ulnar nerve in the forearm via the Martin–Gruber anastomosis, or acts as a conduit for the median nerve to innervate all the lumbricals, not only the first two. The important principle to remember is that when strange patterns of deficits occur following median or ulnar nerve injury, one should consider these potential communications when deciding if an injury is complete or incomplete.

♦ Sensory Innervation

Excluding the medial brachial and antebrachial cutaneous nerves, which originate from the medial cord (described previously), the ulnar nerve has three sensory branches. These branches provide sensory innervation to the medial one third of the hand (**Fig. 2–21**). The *dorsal ulnar cutaneous nerve* pierces the antebrachial fascia just proximal to the dorsomedial wrist. It crosses the wrist and ramifies to innervate the dorsomedial one third of the hand. It also innervates the dorsum of the fifth and medial one half of the fourth digits. The skin under and surrounding the fingernail is innervated however, by the superficial sensory division of the ulnar nerve, whose branches arise from the volar surface. Sensory testing for the dorsal ulnar cutaneous nerve should take place on the dorsal surface of the medial third of the hand.

The *palmar ulnar cutaneous nerve* enters the subcutaneous space of the hypothenar eminence and provides sensory innervation to this area. This nerve innervates the whole medial one third of the palm. Because of sensory territory variations, however, the best area to test this nerve's function is on the hypothenar eminence.

The *superficial sensory division* of the ulnar nerve, besides innervating the palmaris brevis muscle, is a pure sensory nerve. It carries sensation from the volar surface of the fifth and medial one half of the fourth digits, including the dorsal aspect of the distal phalanges. The digital nerves carry sensation from the fingers to the superficial sensory division. The optimal area to test autonomous sensation for this nerve is on the volar aspect of the fifth digit.

- **Frequent variation in sensory territories between these three ulnar branches occurs. For example, the palmar ulnar cutaneous nerve can only cover the proximal hypothenar eminence, with the superficial sensory division covering the remaining medial, volar surface of the palm.**

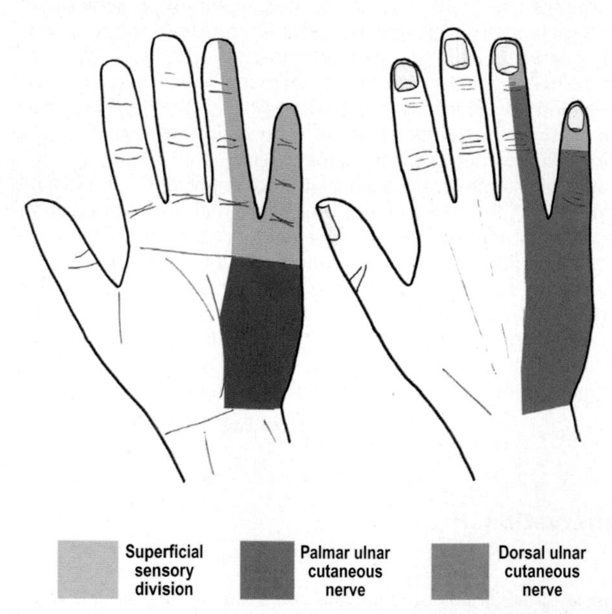

Figure 2–21 Sensory innervation from the ulnar nerve. The ulnar nerve has three sensory branches. These branches provide sensory innervation to the medial one third of the hand.

Another common variation is for the median (more common), or ulnar nerve, to carry all the sensory fibers from the fourth digit.

♦ Clinical Findings and Syndromes

In contrast to the median nerve, where entrapment usually occurs at the wrist and rarely in the proximal forearm/elbow, for the ulnar nerve the opposite is true: It is compressed most commonly at the elbow, and rarely at the wrist.

The Arm

Complete Palsy

Ulnar nerve palsies in the arm region are usually caused by trauma, including gunshot wounds, lacerations, and blunt injuries. Because of its close proximity to the median nerve and brachial artery, concomitant injury to these three structures may occur. As with the median nerve, the ulnar nerve may be compressed by using a crutch or hanging the arm over a chair (*Saturday night palsy*).

A complete ulnar nerve lesion is quite devastating, considering the loss of fine, coordinated hand movements. To begin, a severe ulnar lesion causes loss of sensation in the hypothenar eminence (palmar ulnar cutaneous branch), the volar surface of the fifth and half of the fourth digits (superficial sensory division), and the dorsomedial one third of the hand and fingers (dorsal ulnar cutaneous nerve). However, if sensory abnormalities extend more than 2 cm proximal to the wrist crease one should alternatively consider involvement of the medial antebrachial cutaneous nerve, and therefore the medial cord of the brachial plexus or C8/T1 nerve roots. Regarding motor loss, wrist flexion will be weak and only in a radial direction, from the unopposed contraction of the flexor carpi radialis (median innervated). The distal phalanges of the fourth and especially the fifth digits will not flex secondary to partial flexor digitorum profundus weakness. Marked hand intrinsic weakness occurs, with the only residual function provided by the median nerve innervated thenar muscles. Muscle wasting can eventually be seen, including the hypothenar eminence, the dorsal interosseous muscles, and even the thenar eminence secondary to wasting of the large adductor pollicis muscle. There is loss of finger abduction and adduction, from paralysis of both the dorsal and palmar interossei, respectively. However, as mentioned earlier, some finger abduction or adduction can still occur because of substitution by the long finger extensors and flexors.

Ulnar claw hand is when opening the hand, there is hyperextension at the metacarpal-phalangeal joints in the fourth and especially the fifth digits, along with partial flexion of both interphalangeal joints in these two fingers (**Fig. 2–22**). Ulnar claw hand results from a loss of function in the third and fourth lumbricals, along with paralysis of the interossei and flexor digit minimi, which causes flexion weakness at the metacarpal-phalangeal joints. The extensor digitorum communis (radial nerve) becomes unopposed, thereby placing these two metacarpal-phalangeal joints in hyperextension. Despite paralysis of the flexor digitorum profundus in these two digits, its tendons are still placed on tension. This is because of both finger's hyperextension, as well as from residual tone in this muscle secondary to its median nerve innervated portion. Furthermore, when a severe or complete ulnar nerve lesion occurs distal to the flexor digitorum profundus (i.e., a lesion that spares this muscle), the degree of claw hand is worse because even more unopposed distal

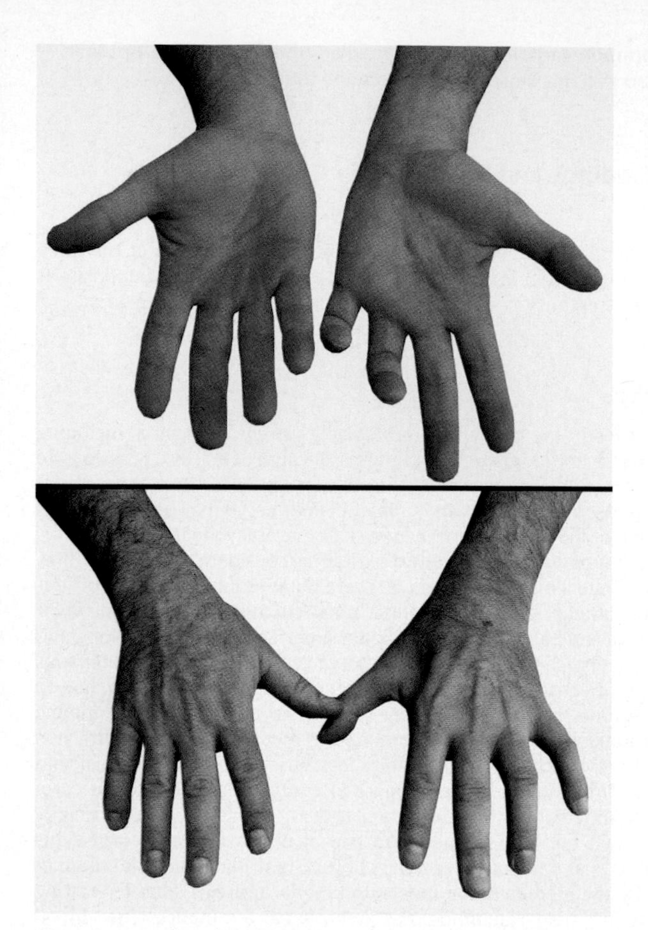

Figure 2–22 Ulnar claw hand (patient's left). The ulnar claw hand occurs when opening the hand, there is hyperextension of the metacarpal-phalangeal joints in the fourth and especially the fifth digits. Both interphalangeal joints are also partially flexed in these two fingers. Atrophy of the first dorsal interosseous muscle is evident on the dorsal view (bottom). The patient's normal right hand is shown for comparison.

finger flexion occurs. Without proper physical therapy, ulnar claw hand may become permanent, secondary to contractures.

Wartenburg's sign is when the fifth digit is slightly more abducted when compared with the normal hand. This occurs because the third palmar interosseous muscle, which adducts the fifth digit, is paralyzed; the unopposed action of the extensor digiti minimi and extensor digitorum communis of the radial nerve causes the finger to rest in a slightly more-abducted position.

Froment's sign can be elicited when the patient is asked to pull apart a piece of paper held between the complete volar surface of each straightened thumb and closed fist (**Fig. 2–23**). In the affected hand, the adductor pollicis is weak and thumb adduction does not occur. Instead, the interphalangeal joint of the

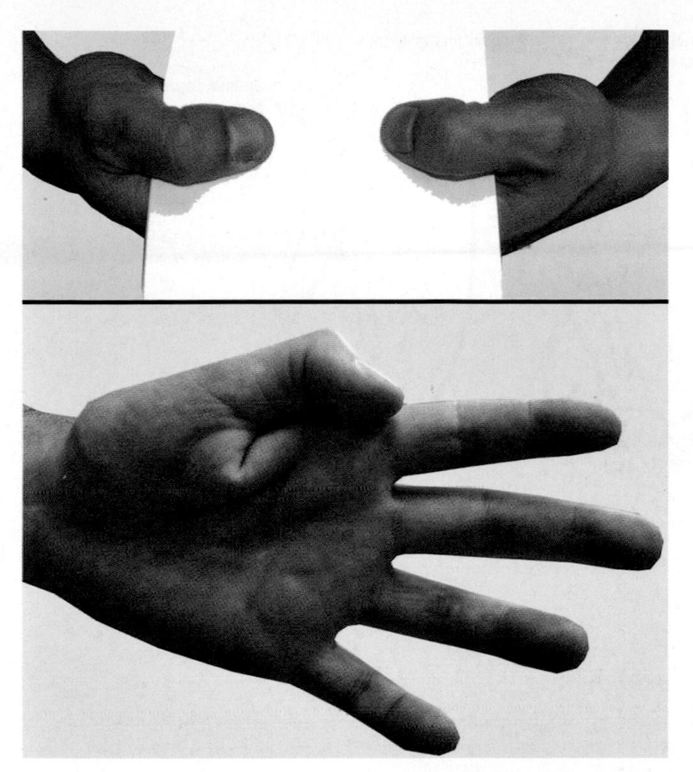

Figure 2–23 Froment's sign. When the adductor pollicis is weak, thumb adduction does not occur. Instead, contraction of the flexor pollicis longus muscle substitutes for this movement by flexing the interphalangeal joint of the thumb. The upper photograph illustrates a bilateral Froment's sign when a subject attempts to pull apart a piece of paper. The lower figure reveals a Froment's sign when the patient is instructed to hold a straightened thumb against the lateral margin of the hand.

affected thumb flexes to hold the paper through contraction of the flexor pollicis longus (median innervated).

Arcade of Struthers

Once piercing the intermuscular septum about halfway down the arm, the ulnar nerve runs along, and slightly within, the medial head of the triceps. In approximately 50% of the population, an arcade of fascia, the arcade of Struthers, extends over the ulnar nerve from the intermuscular septum to the superficial surface of the medial head of the triceps. This arcade is a few centimeters in length and occurs approximately 8 cm proximal to the elbow.

The arcade of Struthers, in fact, does not cause primary ulnar nerve compression. Instead, it has been posited as the reason why some ulnar nerve transpositions at the elbow fail; the arcade of Struthers, when present and not transected during the original transposition surgery, may tether the relocated ulnar nerve, which leads to compression and recurrent symptoms (**Fig. 2–24**).

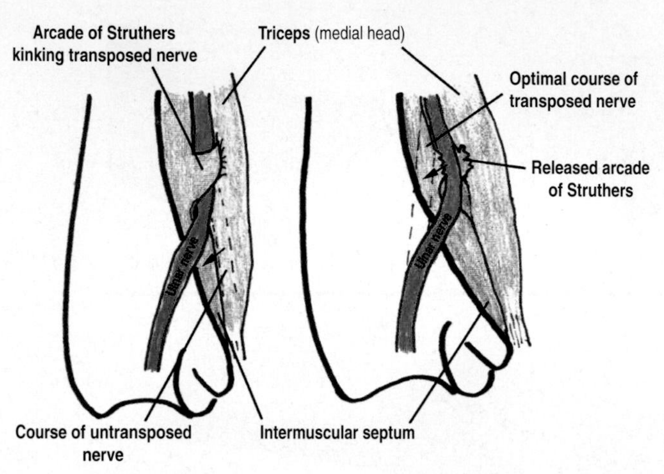

Figure 2–24 Arcade of Struthers compressing a transposed ulnar nerve. It is purported that if this fascial arcade is present and not transected during the original transposition surgery, then a medially transposed nerve at the elbow can become tethered at the arcade of Struthers leading to a new area of compression and recurrent symptoms.

The Elbow

Olecranon Notch

Compression of the ulnar nerve at the elbow is a common entrapment, second only to carpal tunnel syndrome (**Fig. 2–25**). It usually presents with sensory

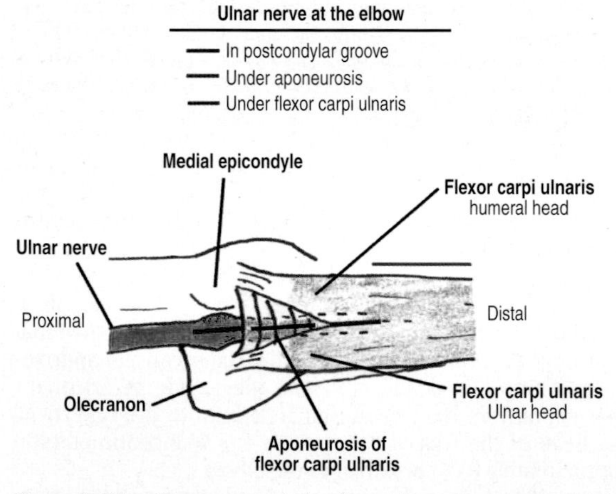

Figure 2–25 Compression at the elbow. The most common point of ulnar nerve damage, as evidenced by intraoperative nerve action potential recordings, is at the postcondylar groove just proximal to its covering aponeurosis. Other points of possible ulnar nerve entrapment at the elbow include between the two heads of the flexor carpi ulnaris (cubital tunnel syndrome), and by Osborne's fascia, when present.

changes in the fifth and fourth digits, including hyperesthesia, hypesthesia, and paresthesias. At first, these symptoms are intermittent, often induced by prolonged forearm flexion or direct compression of the ulnar nerve in the post-condylar grove. Ask about repetitive actions and a history of mild trauma. These sensory symptoms can occur at night if one sleeps with the arm in flexion or if the elbow lies on a hard surface when the forearm is extended and supinated, thus exposing the ulnar nerve to compression. Although not as common as with carpal tunnel syndrome, symptoms from ulnar nerve compression at the elbow can also wake the patient up at night. Abnormal light touch and vibration sense may be evident on examination. Provocative maneuvers, like flexing the forearm for a minute, may precipitate symptoms. The patient should also repetitively flex the elbow while you palpate the ulnar nerve in the postcondylar groove to rule out "snapping" or dislocation of either the ulnar nerve or medial triceps tendon, both of which can cause ulnar nerve irritation at the elbow. One must keep in mind, however, that the majority of patients with prolapsing ulnar nerves are asymptomatic.

As nerve damage progresses, patients usually report numbness that is more persistent. They report pain in the postcondylar region often radiating down the medial forearm to the hand. A Tinel's sign at the postcondylar groove may be present. With more nerve damage, patients begin to have weakness in the ulnar innervated hand intrinsic muscles. They may report clumsiness with fine hand movements, like buttoning buttons or using a pen. With moderate to severe damage, two-point discrimination can also be affected. To ascertain subtle hand intrinsic weakness, one can observe the following finger movements: rapid thumb to fingertip touching (observe slowing and lack of precision), synchronous digit flexion and extension (look for early claw hand), and if available, power grip testing (usually decreased up to 80% with ulnar palsies).

With more severe and chronic compression, persistent numbness, hand intrinsic weakness, ulnar nerve tenderness at the elbow, and muscular atrophy may be present. When atrophy occurs, it is most readily noted at the hypothenar eminence and first dorsal interosseous muscle. Median nerve innervated hand intrinsics (e.g., abductor pollicis brevis) should be normal, or else a C8/T1 spinal nerve/lower trunk lesion may be present (e.g., neurogenic thoracic outlet syndrome). Ulnar claw hand, Wartenberg's sign, and Froment's sign are all usually present in severe, chronic cases. Despite branches to the flexor carpi ulnaris often originating from the ulnar nerve distal to the post-condylar groove, weakness of this muscle in cubital tunnel syndrome is rare. This has been attributed to the fact that the sensory and hand intrinsic fibers in the ulnar nerve at the elbow are more superficial, and perhaps, more prone to irritation. If flexor carpi ulnaris weakness is present or occurs early in the presentation, a lesion more proximal to the postcondylar groove should be considered.

The most common point of ulnar nerve damage, as evidenced by intraoperative nerve action potential recordings, is at the postcondylar groove just proximal to its covering aponeurosis. Other points of possible ulnar nerve entrapment at the elbow include between the two heads of the flexor carpi ulnaris (cubital tunnel syndrome) and by Osborne's fascia, when present.

- **Tardive ulnar palsy refers to a person with late-onset ulnar nerve compression at the elbow following an elbow fracture years earlier. In these patients, the fracture causes a capitus valgus deformity at the elbow (with the elbow extended, the forearm is not straight in relation to the** humerus, but instead angles laterally). This anatomical situation increases tension on the medially located ulnar nerve (by increasing the distance it must travel), thereby predisposing it to compression at the elbow. On a separate note, the anconeus muscle, which runs between the medial epicondyle and olecranon in some patients, may also cause ulnar nerve entrapment at the elbow. The most frequent operative positioning injury affects the ulnar nerve at the elbow.

The Forearm

Flexor-Pronator Fascia

Although exceedingly rare, the ulnar nerve may be irritated by a thickened flexor-pronator fascia. Compression by this structure would occur in the proximal to mid-forearm (approximately 5 cm distal to the medial epicondyle), where the ulnar nerve passes between the flexor carpi ulnaris and the flexor-pronator muscle mass. The fascia of this latter muscle mass may be excessively thickened, thereby predisposing one to compression. Although a clear syndrome has not been reported, repetitive forearm pronation and wrist flexion is thought to be associated with this form of compression.

The Dorsal Ulnar Cutaneous Nerve

Occasionally, the dorsal ulnar cutaneous branch may be compressed or transected as it leaves the ulnar nerve and passes to the dorsum of the wrist between the flexor carpi ulnaris tendon and the ulna. Ulnar fractures or repairs, lacerations, and/or blunt trauma may be causative. The patient presents with numbness or hypesthesia in the dorsomedial one third of the hand in this branch's anatomical distribution. With some lesions, a Tinel's sign can be elicited when tapping on the medial border of the ulna approximately 5 cm proximal to the wrist.

The Wrist

Guyon's Tunnel

Ulnar nerve compression at the wrist is rare. Nonetheless, based on the ulnar nerve's branching pattern in Guyon's tunnel, three "zones" of compression have been described: zone, compression of the ulnar nerve prior to its division in Guyon's tunnel; zone 2, compression of only the deep motor division; and zone 3, compression of only the superficial sensory division (**Fig. 2–26**).

Zone 1 lesions affect the ulnar nerve before it divides. The etiology is usually a fracture or ganglion cyst compressing the nerve in the proximal two thirds of Guyon's tunnel. Sensory loss occurs on the volar surfaces of the fifth and medial half of the fourth fingers, including the nail beds. Sensation to the hypothenar eminence is commonly spared because the palmar ulnar cutaneous nerve is unaffected. Patients with zone 1 compression can have intrinsic hand muscle weakness including a claw hand, Wartenberg's sign, and Froment's sign. The claw hand can be quite severe because innervation to the flexor digitorum profundus is preserved.

Zone 2 lesions compress only the deep motor branch, and therefore no sensory loss occurs. The motor deficits are similar to a zone 1 lesion. To confirm that the superficial sensory division is intact, one may check for a *palmaris brevis sign*, which is simply observing the contraction of the palmaris brevis (**Fig. 2–12**). Innervation of this small muscle is from the proximal superficial sensory division, and therefore if this muscle contracts, one knows that this division is at

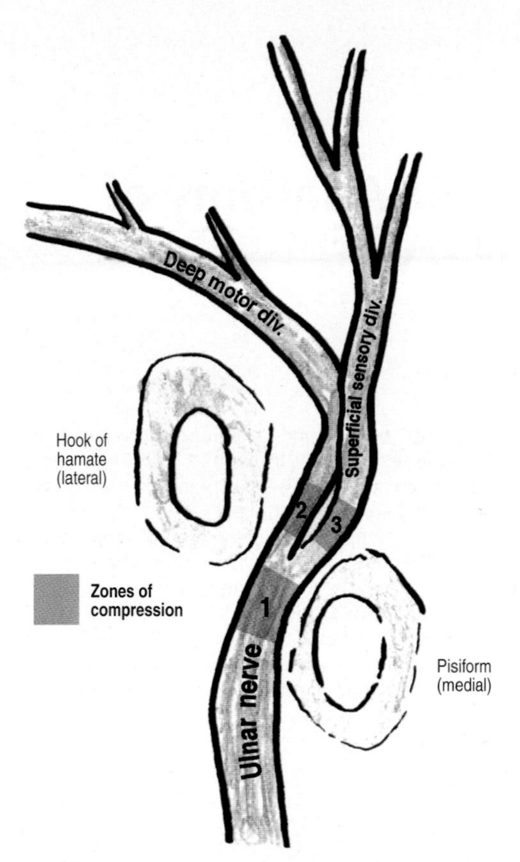

Figure 2–26 Zones of compression in Guyon's tunnel. Based on the ulnar nerve's branching pattern in Guyon's tunnel, three "zones" of compression have been described: zone 1, compression of the ulnar nerve prior to its division in Guyon's tunnel (most common); zone 2, compression of only the deep motor branch; and zone 3, compression of only the superficial sensory division (least common).

least partially functioning. Zone 2 lesions are usually caused by ganglion cysts. Occasionally, just the hypothenar branch from the deep motor division is injured, causing isolated weakness of the hypothenar muscles.

Zone 3 lesions affect only the superficial sensory division, and are the least common variety of ulnar entrapment at the wrist. A reliable area to test for sensory loss is on the volar surface of the fifth digit. All motor function is usually spared and the palmaris brevis sign may be absent (no contraction). A distal ulnar artery thrombosis or aneurysm may be causative.

Ulnar nerve compression at the wrist can also be secondary to direct pressure. This can occur from prolonged writing, using a computer or mouse, and from riding a bicycle. These lesions present with a combination of motor and sensory symptoms and usually respond well to conservative treatment.

3

The Diagnostic Anatomy of the Radial Nerve

The radial nerve is the "great extensor" of the upper arm, innervating nearly all the extensor movements in the upper extremity. Although its chief importance is muscular innervation, the radial nerve also carries sensory information from a significant portion of the posterior arm, forearm, and hand.

More so than for any other nerve, a complete understanding of radial nerve palsies and entrapment syndromes requires mastery of its three-dimensional (3D) anatomy. This is because, in contrast to the median and ulnar nerves, whose paths are relatively linear and uncomplicated, the radial nerve spirals its way down the arm, back and forth between the flexor and extensor compartments. Most importantly, one must understand the location, origins, and insertions of the triceps and supinator muscles, which are intimately related to the radial nerve.

♦ Anatomical Course

The Axilla

After giving off the thoracodorsal and axillary nerve branches, the posterior cord of the brachial plexus continues distally as the radial nerve. The radial nerve is the largest terminal branch from the brachial plexus. It is made up of the C5 to C8 nerve roots. The radial nerve is located posterior to the axillary artery in the axilla. This relationship with the axillary artery is in contrast to the median and ulnar nerves, both of which are located more anteriorly.

In the distal axilla and proximal arm, the radial nerve drifts further posterior to the brachial artery. As with the other brachial plexus branches, the radial nerve is located, deep to the pectoralis major and minor, when it exits the axilla, the radial nerve lies superficial to three sequential muscles, which together constitute the posterior axillobrachial border (from proximal to distal): (1) the subscapularis muscle that inserts into the humeral head, (2) the latissimus dorsi tendon that inserts into both the head and surgical neck of the humerus, and shortly thereafter, (3) the teres major that inserts into the surgical neck of the humerus (**Fig. 3–1**). In the proximal upper arm, the radial nerve continues distally by running on the anterior surface of the long head of the triceps, a muscle that originates in the axilla from the lateral scapula.

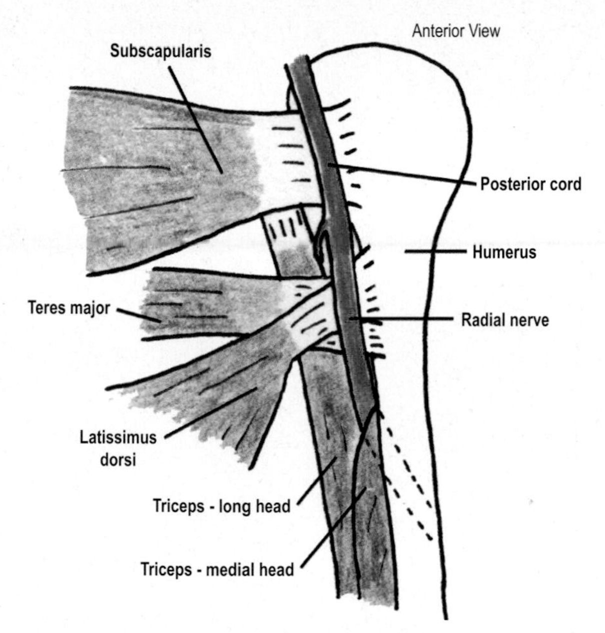

Figure 3–1 Radial nerve in the distal axilla. The radial nerve lies superficial to three sequential muscles as it exits the axilla (from proximal to distal): the subscapularis muscle that inserts into the humeral head; the latissimus dorsi tendon that inserts into both the head and surgical neck of the humerus; and the teres major that inserts into the surgical neck of the humerus. The radial nerve enters the arm upon (superficial to) the long head of the triceps, and almost immediately dives into the cleft between the long and medial triceps' heads. Within this cleft, the nerve runs toward the most proximal portion of the spiral groove.

♦ **In approximately 10% of the population, the radial nerve also carries fibers from the T1 spinal nerve.**

The Axilla to the Spiral Groove

The triceps has three heads—the long, medial, and lateral—all of which share a common insertion upon the olecranon, and act in unison to extend the forearm. Their names are derived from their respective origins. The long head is so named because it goes all the way from the scapula, high in the axilla, down to the olecranon. It has a relatively straight course between these two points. The medial head of the triceps originates along the medial and posterior humeral shaft, remains anterior and medial to the long head of the triceps, and posterior and medial to the humerus. The lateral head originates along the lateral shaft of the humerus, and remains lateral to both the long head of the triceps and the humerus. These origins of the lateral and medial heads of the triceps run parallel along the humerus in a spiral fashion (**Fig. 3–2**). This spiral insertion begins posteromedially, and curves distally by running posterior, then lateral, along the humerus. The thin, bare area of bone between the origins of the lateral and medial heads of the triceps is called the *spiral groove*.

After entering the arm on (superficial to) the long head of the triceps, the radial nerve almost immediately dives into the cleft between the long and

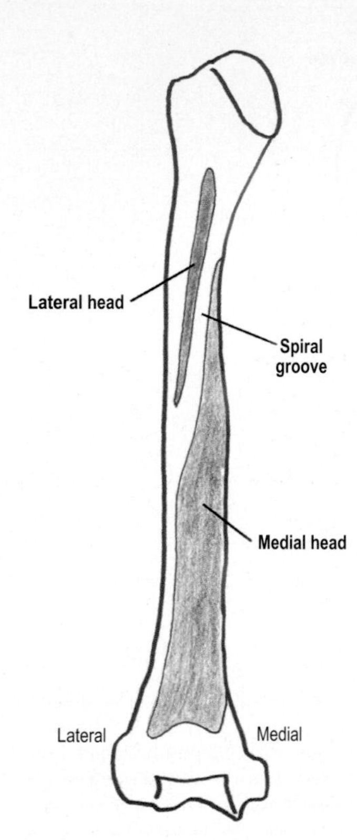

Figure 3–2 Origin of medial and lateral heads of the triceps on the humerus (posterior view). The origins of these heads of the triceps run parallel along the humerus in a spiral fashion. This spiral begins posteromedially, and curves distally by running posterior, then lateral, along the humerus.

medial triceps' heads (**Fig. 3–1**). The brachial profunda artery runs with the radial nerve in this cleft. Together they course posteriorly and medially toward the most proximal portion of the spiral groove. Once reaching the spiral groove, the radial nerve continues distally by running posterior and lateral to the humerus between the origins of the lateral and medial heads of the triceps (i.e., along the spiral groove). The nerve remains in contact with the humerus and is covered by the lateral head of the triceps until it pierces the lateral intermuscular septum, about halfway down the arm, just distal to the deltoid's insertion into the humerus.

The Spiral Groove to the Supinator Muscle

Just distal to the spiral groove, the radial nerve enters the flexor compartment by piercing the lateral intermuscular septum. At this point the radial nerve is quite immobile and superficial, and therefore prone to injury. Once in the flexor compartment, from mid-arm to antecubital fossa, the radial nerve runs underneath the following three muscles, which sequentially arcade over the nerve: (1) the brachioradialis, (2) the extensor carpi radialis longus, and (3) the extensor carpi radialis brevis (**Fig. 3–3**). This anatomical arrangement has been referred to as the *radial tunnel*. The last muscle, the extensor carpi radialis brevis, is unique in that it originates underneath the nerve, but subsequently loops over it; an anatomical arrangement that can predispose to nerve irritation. In this region,

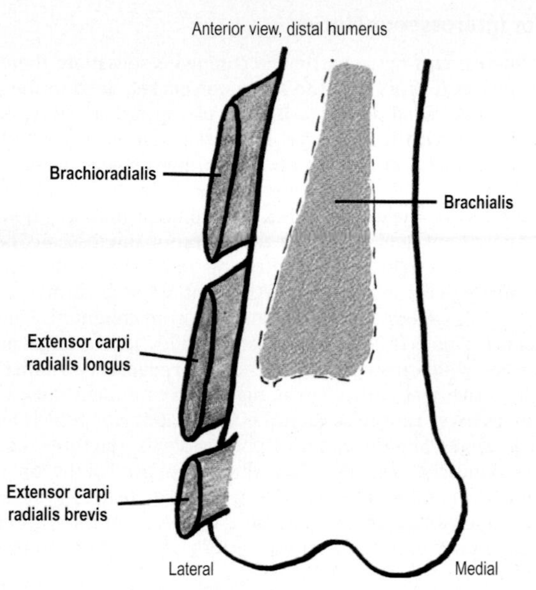

Figure 3–3 Upon entering the flexor compartment at mid-arm level, the radial nerve runs underneath three muscles, which sequentially arcade over the nerve. This anatomical arrangement has been referred to as the *radial tunnel*. The origins of these muscles are depicted.

the brachialis muscle lies medial and posterior to the radial nerve and the lateral epicondyle of the humerus is posterior to the radial nerve.

Distal to the elbow joint, the radial nerve lies on the most proximal portion of the supinator muscle's deep head (see below). In this area, the radial nerve bifurcates into the posterior interosseous and superficial sensory radial nerves. The location of this bifurcation is quite variable, and can be either proximal or distal to the lateral epicondyle.

Allow your right arm to hang at your side in anatomical position (supinated). Grasp your right forearm with your left hand, just distal to the lateral epicondyle, so that the web space between your thumb and index finger is on the lateral border of the arm with your fingertips pointed in the direction of the elbow joint. Your left hand is the supinator muscle. The supinator muscle originates from the anterior, lateral, and posterior aspects of the radial bone (your palm), and attaches more proximally to the anterior and lateral portions of the lateral epicondyle of the humerus (thumb tip), as well as to the most superior portion of the ulna's posterior surface (fingertips). As the forearm pronates with an extended elbow, the supinator muscle is stretched as the radius crosses anterior to the ulna. With subsequent supinator contraction, and resultant shortening of this muscle, the arm supinates.

This muscle has both a deep and superficial head. If you had two left hands and put the second one on top of the first, it would replicate the anatomical relationship between these two heads. The radial nerve has a characteristic relationship to the supinator muscle. The superficial head of this muscle forms a "pocket," like on a pair of jeans, into which the posterior interosseous nerve descends. The edge of this pocket can be fibrous and is termed the *arcade of Frohse*. The superficial sensory radial nerve remains superficial to the superficial head of the supinator.

The Posterior Interosseous Nerve

The posterior interosseous nerve carries no cutaneous sensation; therefore, it is a "pure" motor nerve. It dives into the supinator pocket, deep to the arcade of Frohse. The recurrent radial artery, a branch of the radial artery, enters the supinator's "pocket" with the posterior interosseous nerve. Once between the two heads of the supinator muscle, the posterior interosseous nerve travels laterally around the head of the radius, entering the extensor compartment of the forearm. In some people, the deep head of the supinator muscle is quite thin, or occasionally even absent, and therefore the posterior interosseous nerve may actually lie directly on the radius. After emerging from between the two heads of the supinator muscle in the extensor compartment of the forearm, the posterior interosseous nerve lies deep to the extensor digitorum communis, and superficial to the abductor pollicis longus. It then ramifies into a large number of unnamed branches, which are often called the *cauda equina of the arm* **(Fig. 3–4).** While remaining underneath the extensor digitorum communis muscle, the posterior interosseous nerve runs in sequence over the abductor pollicis longus, the extensor pollicis longus, and the extensor pollicis brevis (the three radial nerve-innervated thumb muscles). Distally, along the bottom third of the forearm, some of the branches of the posterior interosseous nerve are quite deep, lying directly on (posterior to) the interosseous membrane. Here, the posterior interosseous artery, a branch from the interosseous communis artery, which stems from the ulnar artery, joins them.

The Superficial Sensory Radial Nerve

This terminal division of the radial nerve remains superficial to the supinator muscle, but deep to the brachioradialis muscle. In fact, it remains underneath the brachioradialis muscle until approximately two thirds of the way down the forearm (**Fig. 3–5**), running on the posterior (deep) muscular bed of the extensor carpi radialis longus. More distally, but still proximal to the wrist, the tendons of these two muscles form and separate, with the brachioradialis tendon more anterior and the extensor carpi radialis longus tendon more posterior. Between

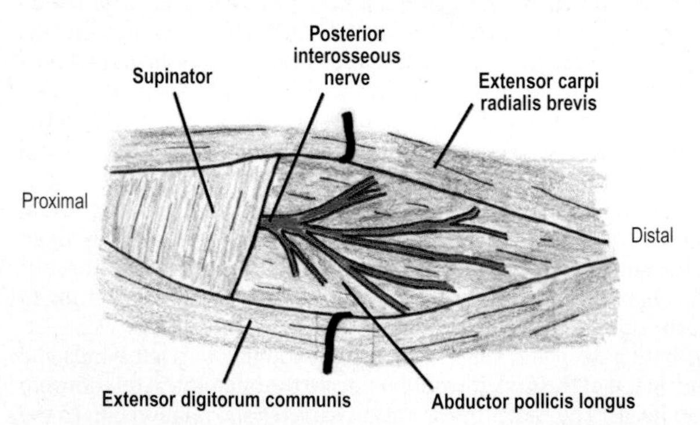

Figure 3–4 Once emerging from between the two heads of the supinator muscle in the extensor compartment of the dorsal forearm, the posterior interosseous nerve lies deep to the extensor digitorum communis, and superficial to the abductor pollicis longus. It then ramifies into a large number of unnamed branches, which are often called the *cauda equina of the arm*.

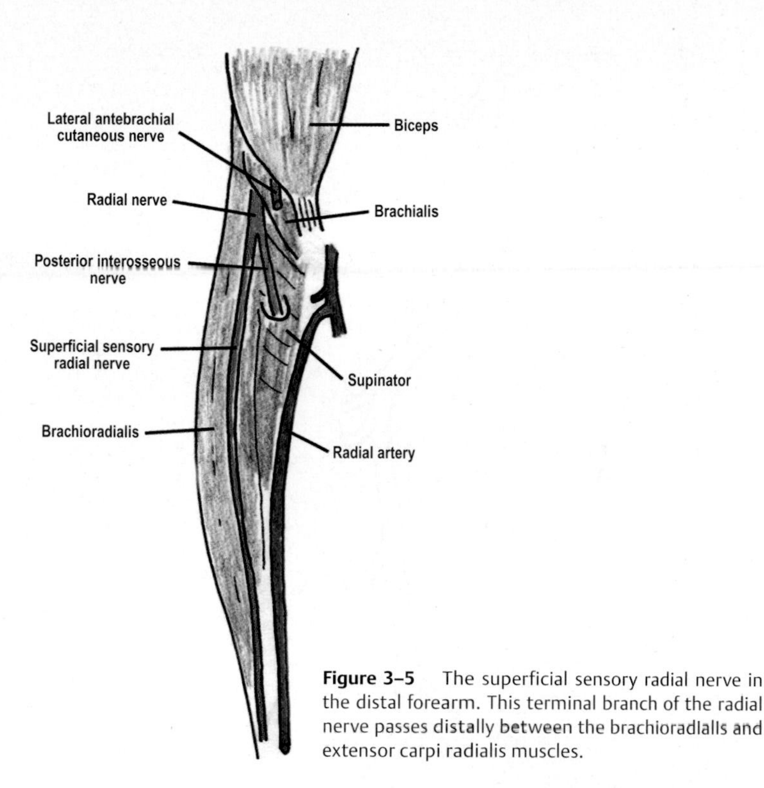

Figure 3–5 The superficial sensory radial nerve in the distal forearm. This terminal branch of the radial nerve passes distally between the brachioradlalls and extensor carpi radialis muscles.

this "fork" in the tendons, and on the lateral edge of the radius, the superficial sensory radial nerve pierces the antebrachial fascia to become subcutaneous. This nerve then passes to the dorsal aspect of the wrist, and branches upon the dorsolateral aspect of the hand, superficial to the extensor retinaculum. The superficial sensory radial nerve usually has four or more terminal branches.

♦ Motor Innervation and Testing

As the great extensor of the upper extremity, the radial nerve innervates four groups of muscles: the triceps group (one muscle, three heads), the lateral epicondyle group (four muscles), the posterior interosseous nerve-superficial group (three muscles), and the posterior interosseous nerve-deep group (four muscles) (**Fig. 3–6**).

The Triceps Group

The long head of the triceps is the first muscle innervated by the radial nerve. Fibers to this muscle arise very proximally at the axillobrachial junction. The next muscle to be innervated is the medial triceps head, followed by the lateral triceps head. This pattern of innervation is logical considering the sequence of

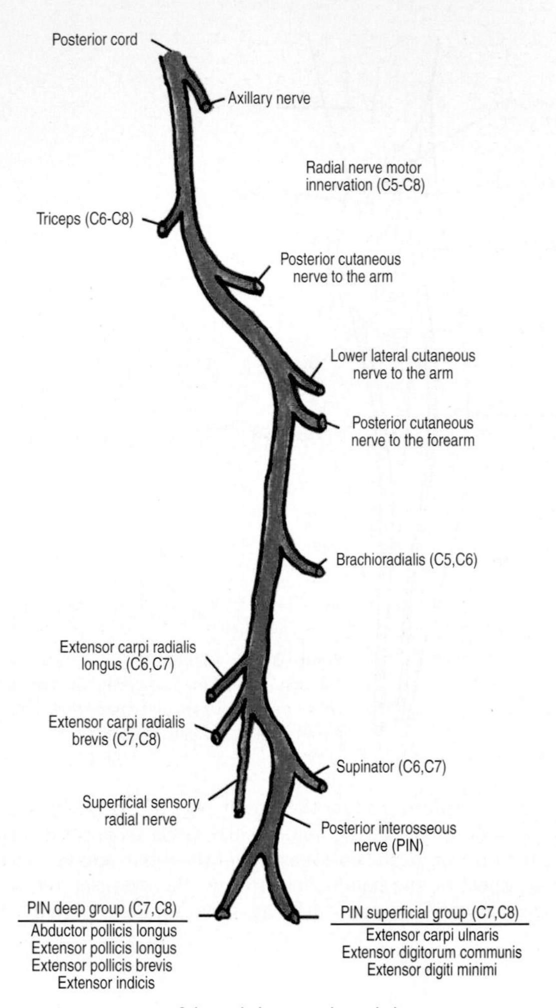

Figure 3–6 Motor innervation of the radial nerve. The radial nerve innervates muscles that extend the forearm, hand, and fingers. It also supinates and flexes the forearm.

contact between the radial nerve and the three heads of the triceps. The main branches to the medial and lateral heads originate proximal to where the radial nerve enters the spiral groove. However, additional branches to these two muscles arise directly from the radial nerve in the spiral groove. To test the *triceps* (C6-C8), have the patient start by placing the upper arm parallel to the ground, which eliminates the effect of gravity. With the forearm half-extended, support the limb at the elbow and instruct the patient to extend the forearm fully against resistance (**Fig. 3–7**).

- **In 50% of the population, the lateral head of the triceps is innervated prior to the medial head.**

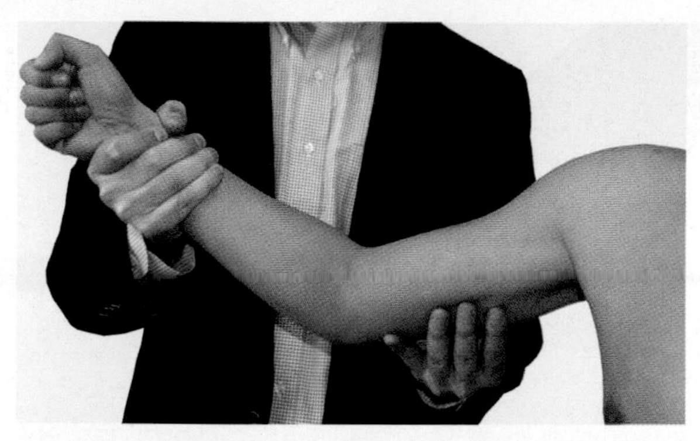

Figure 3–7 Triceps muscle (C6-C8) assessment: Have the patient place the upper arm parallel to the ground, which eliminates the effect of gravity. Starting with the forearm half-extended, support the limb at the elbow and instruct the patient to fully extend the forearm against resistance.

The Lateral Epicondyle Group

All branches to the *brachioradialis* (C5, C6) originate from the radial nerve proximal to the lateral epicondyle. To test this muscle, have the patient flex the forearm against resistance with the forearm halfway between pronation and supination (**Fig. 3–8**). With contraction, the brachioradialis muscle becomes prominent in the lateral antecubital fossa, where it can be observed and palpated.

The two more distal muscles, the *extensor carpi radialis longus* (C6, C7) *and brevis* (C7, C8) are assessed together by having the patient extend and abduct (bend radially) the hand against resistance (**Fig. 3–9**), while you stabilize the distal forearm with your other hand. With the arm pronated, these muscle bellies can be seen lateral to the brachioradialis. Most branches to the extensor carpi radialis longus originate from the radial nerve above the lateral epicondyle, while branches to the extensor carpi radialis brevis originate below the lateral epicondyle.

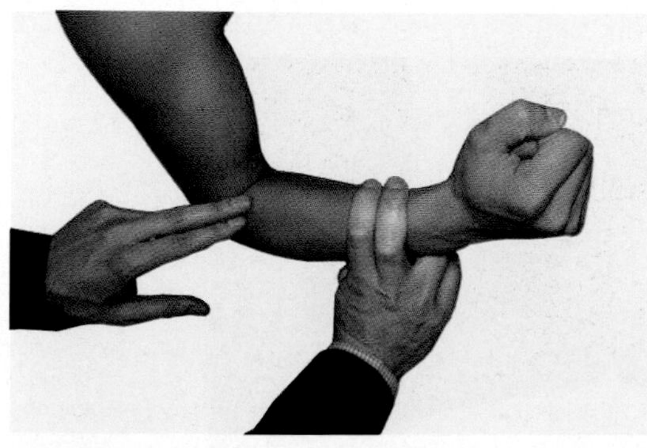

Figure 3–8 Brachioradialis (C5, C6) assessment: The patient flexes at the elbow with the forearm halfway between pronation and supination. With contraction, the brachioradialis muscle becomes prominent in the lateral antecubital fossa, where it can be observed and palpated.

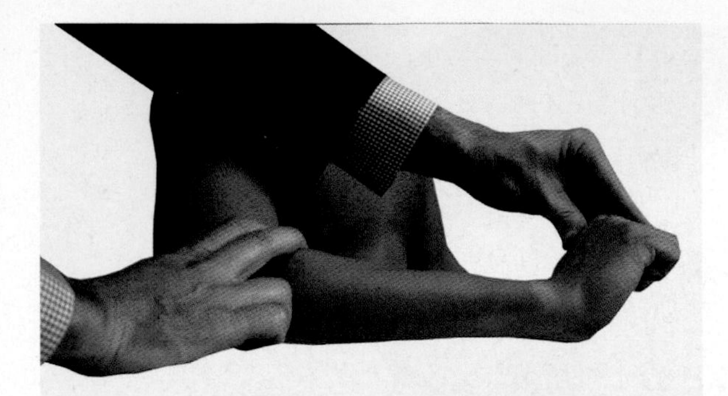

Figure 3–9 Extensor carpi radialis longus (C6, C7) and brevis (C7, C8) assessment: These two muscles are assessed together by having the patient extend and abduct (bend radially) the hand against resistance. With the arm pronated, contraction of these muscles can be seen lateral to the brachioradialis.

Distal to the lateral epicondyle in the proximal forearm, the posterior interosseous nerve innervates the *supinator* (C6, C7). Branches destined for this muscle originate from the posterior interosseous nerve prior to it passing into the muscle. The supinator muscle supinates the forearm. Although the biceps brachii is also a strong forearm supinator, it can be placed at a mechanical disadvantage by extending the forearm. Therefore, to isolate the supinator it should be tested with the forearm extended (**Fig. 3–10**).

♦ **Because the radial nerve's point of bifurcation into the posterior interosseous and superficial sensory radial nerves is variable, the axons destined for the extensor carpi radialis brevis can originate from the radial nerve proper, or from one of these two distal branches. The brachialis muscle receives some innervation from the radial nerve in this region (in addition to its main innervation from the musculocutaneous nerve). However, this innervation to the brachialis is usually not enough to flex the arm in the presence of musculocutaneous nerve palsy.**

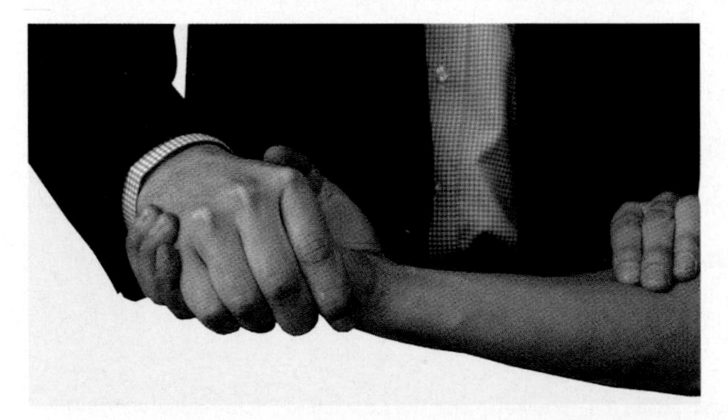

Figure 3–10 Supinator (C6, C7) assessment: The supinator should be tested with the forearm extended, to minimize substitution by the biceps brachii. The patient maintains the forearm in supination as you attempt to pronate it.

The Posterior Interosseous Nerve

The Superficial Group

After passing through the supinator and entering the extensor compartment, the posterior interosseous nerve supplies the superficial group of extensor muscles. This group is made up of the extensor carpi ulnaris, the extensor digitorum communis, and the extensor digiti minimi, which are often supplied by a common branch. Test the *extensor carpi ulnaris* (C7, C8) by stabilizing the distal forearm and having the patient extend and adduct (bend in the ulnar direction) the hand (**Fig. 3–11**). This muscle's tendon at the wrist can be seen and felt. The *extensor digitorum communis* (C7, C8) extends the second to fifth digits at the metacarpal-phalangeal (knuckle) joints. To evaluate this muscle, each finger is extended at the knuckle joint with the forearm and hand well supported in a neutral position. The second (index finger) and fifth digits (small finger) have supplementary extensors, the extensor indicis and digiti minimi, respectively, while the third and fourth do not. Apply resistance just proximal to the proximal interphalangeal joint. The distal finger joints are allowed to relax in flexion (**Fig. 3–12**). Another way to test finger extension at the knuckle joint is to have the patient put his or

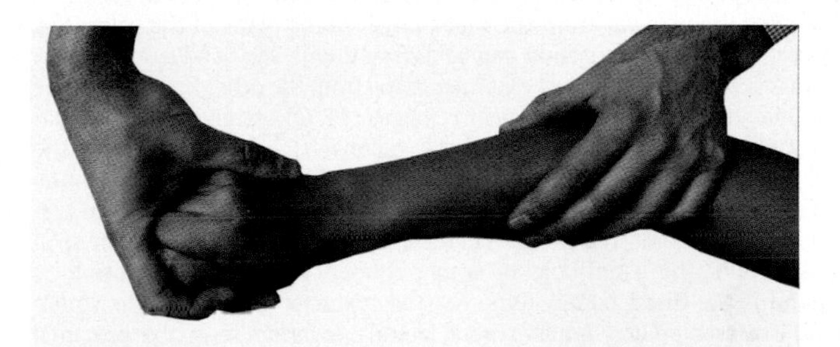

Figure 3–11 Extensor carpi ulnaris (C7, C8) assessment: Test by stabilizing the distal forearm and having the patient extend and adduct (bend in an ulnar direction) the hand. This muscle's tendon at the wrist's edge can be seen and felt.

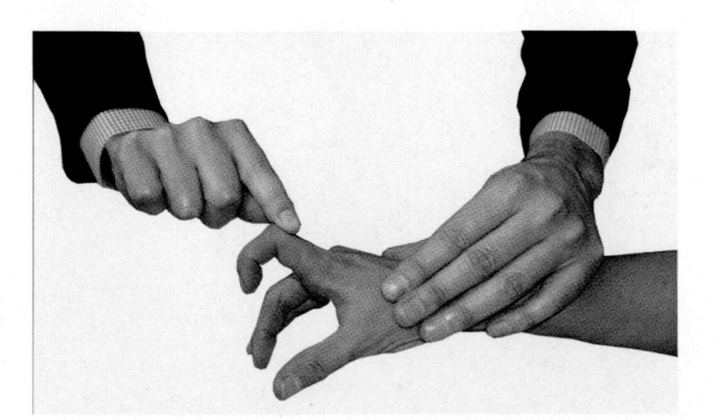

Figure 3–12 Extensor digitorum communis (C7, C8) assessment: To evaluate this muscle, each finger is extended at the knuckle joint with the forearm and hand well supported in a neutral position. Resistance is applied just proximal to the proximal interphalangeal joint. The distal finger joints are allowed to relax in flexion.

her hand and wrist on a flat surface and ask them to extend the fingers either together or individually. The patient should not be allowed to simultaneously flex at the wrist because in doing so, the fingers will extend secondary to tenodesis (i.e., passive movement of a distal joint by changing the distance that a tendon travels by flexing or extending a more proximal joint). The *extensor digiti minimi* (C7, C8) acts in similar fashion as the extensor digitorum communis, yet only upon the fifth digit (**Fig. 3–13**). Keep in mind this digit is normally quite weak and should be compared with the normal hand.

The Deep Group

The deep extensor compartment group may be innervated by separate branches (more common), or it may be innervated via a common ("descending") branch from the posterior interosseous nerve, and include muscles that act upon the thumb and forefinger: the abductor pollicis longus, the extensor pollicis longus, the extensor pollicis brevis, and the extensor indicis. These are the most distally innervated radial muscles, and therefore are the last to be reinnervated following radial nerve injury. The *abductor pollicis longus* (C7, C8) acts to abduct the thumb in a radial direction (in the plane of the palm), unlike the median innervated abductor pollicis brevis, which primarily controls palmar abduction of the thumb. Therefore, one should test the abductor pollicis longus by stabilizing the hand and having the patient move an already extended thumb away from the index finger in the plane of the palm (**Fig. 3–14**). Alternatively, thumb extension can be assessed with the hand as a fist, resting on its ulnar surface. The thumb is extended away from the other fingers, as if the patient was hitchhiking. The *extensor pollicis longus* (C7, C8) extends the interphalangeal joint (**Fig. 3–15**); the *extensor pollicis brevis* (C7, C8) extends at the metacarpal-phalangeal joint (**Fig. 3–16**). This can be remembered by thinking of the extensor pollicis *longus* versus the extensor pollicis *brevis*: the "longer" of the two crosses the more distal joint. The tendons of these three thumb muscles can be seen and palpated around the "snuff box" or scaphoid bone. The sole extensor pollicis longus tendon is the distal border, whereas the abductor pollicis longus (more medial) and extensor pollicis brevis (more lateral), together form the proximal tendinous border. The *extensor indicis* (C7, C8) acts only upon the index finger, and is examined like the extensor digitorum communis (**Fig. 3–12**).

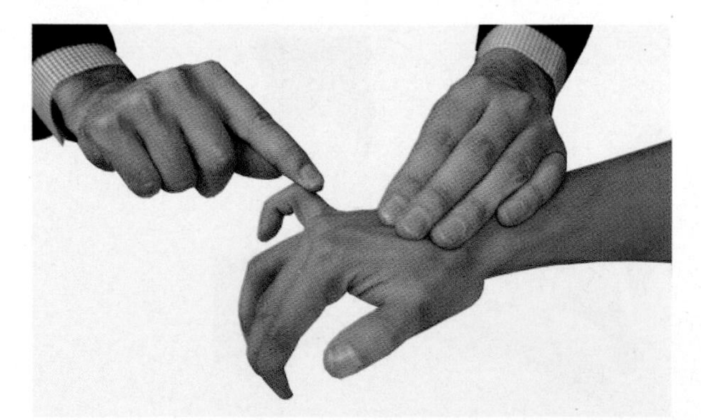

Figure 3–13 Extensor digiti minimi (C7, C8) assessment: This muscle acts in similar fashion as the extensor digitorum communis, yet only upon the fifth digit. The fifth digit is extended at the metacarpal–phalangeal joint while its distal interphalangeal joints are relaxed in flexion.

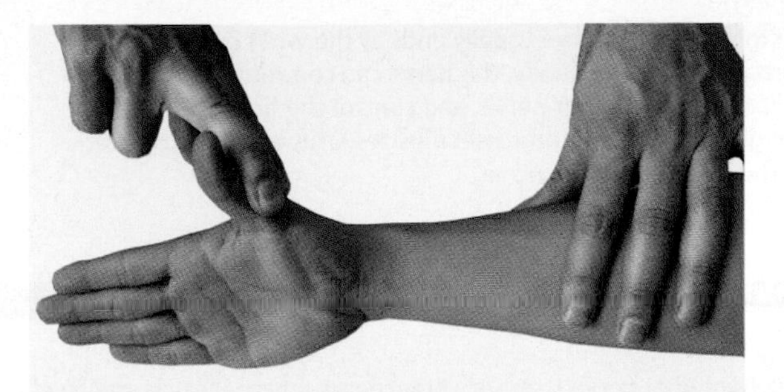

Figure 3–14 Abductor pollicis longus (C7, C8) assessment: This muscle abducts the thumb in a radial direction (in the plane of the palm), unlike the median innervated abductor pollicis brevis, which controls palmar abduction of the thumb. Therefore, one should test the abductor pollicis longus by stabilizing the hand and having the patient move an extended thumb away from the index finger in the plane of the palm.

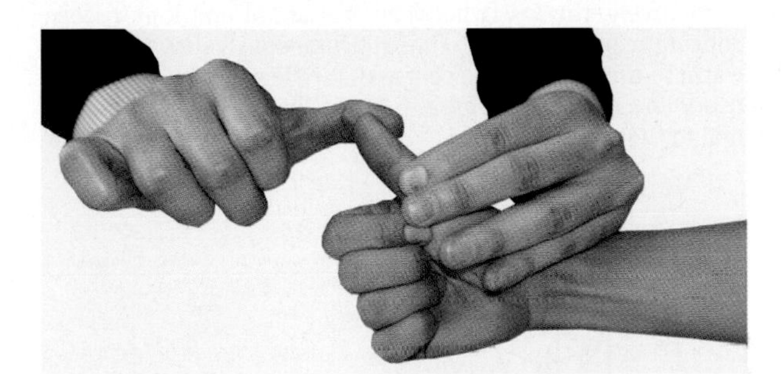

Figure 3–15 Extensor pollicis longus (C7, C8) assessment: Thumb extension is best assessed with the hand as a fist, resting on its ulnar surface. The thumb is extended away from the other fingers, as if the patient is hitchhiking. Resistance is applied to the *distal* phalange to assess the extensor pollicis longus muscle.

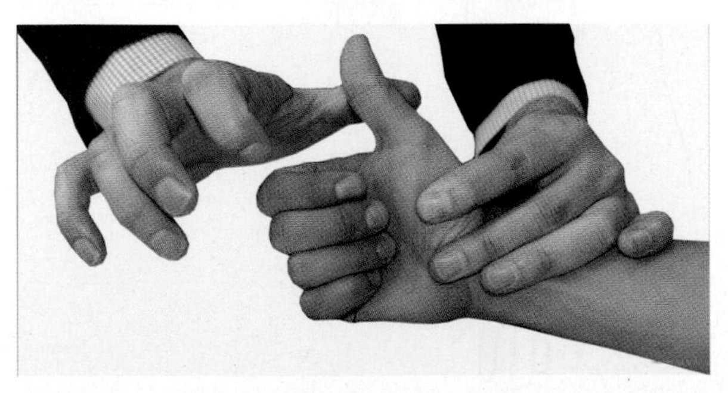

Figure 3–16 Extensor pollicis brevis (C7, C8) assessment: Thumb extension is best assessed with the hand as a fist, resting on its ulnar surface. The thumb is extended away from the other fingers, as if the patient is hitchhiking. Resistance is applied to the *proximal* phalange to assess the extensor pollicis brevis muscle.

- The posterior interosseous nerve usually ends at the wrist by innervating the dorsal carpal bone joints. Rarely, this nerve can communicate with the deep motor branch of the ulnar nerve, and control the first (and perhaps the first through third) dorsal interossei muscles. This anomalous extension is called the *Froment-Rauber nerve*.

♦ Sensory Innervation

Deficits involving the radial nerve's sensory branches can help localize the level of injury. These sensory territories are depicted in **Fig. 3–17.**

The Posterior Cutaneous Nerve to the Arm

The posterior cutaneous nerve to the arm is the first sensory branch from the radial nerve. It originates in the axilla, passes distally with the radial nerve between the long and medial heads of the triceps, and then pierces the lateral triceps head, or, alternatively, the fascia between the lateral and long triceps heads, to become subcutaneous. This nerve runs subcutaneously down the posterior aspect of the arm to the olecranon, a course that reflects its sensory territory. Therefore, sensory loss in the posterior arm is usually indicative of a radial nerve lesion proximal to the spiral groove.

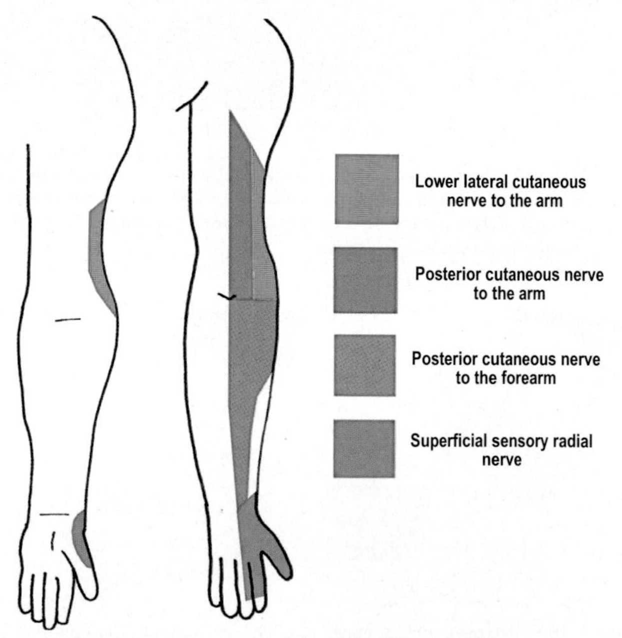

Figure 3–17 Radial nerve sensory branches. The radial nerve carries sensation from the posterior arm, lower lateral arm, posterior forearm, and dorsomedial surface of the hand. Deficits involving these sensory branches can help localize the level of radial nerve injury.

The Lower Lateral Cutaneous Nerve to the Arm

The lower lateral cutaneous nerve to the arm originates from the radial nerve in the spiral groove, and subsequently pierces the brachial fascia at the lateral intermuscular septum to become subcutaneous. This branch's sensory territory includes the lower lateral arm below the deltoid. Sensory loss in this territory, with preserved posterior arm sensation, points toward a radial nerve injury in the spiral groove.

The Posterior Cutaneous Nerve to the Forearm

The posterior cutaneous nerve to the forearm branches from the radial nerve in the brachial-axillary angle, proximal to the origin of the lower lateral cutaneous nerve to the arm. The posterior cutaneous nerve to the forearm runs with the radial nerve in the spiral groove, and then pierces the brachial fascia with the lower lateral cutaneous nerve to the arm at the lateral intermuscular septum. Once subcutaneous, the posterior cutaneous nerve to the forearm passes posterior to the lateral epicondyle, and lateral to the olecranon. Its sensory territory includes the dorsolateral aspect of the forearm.

The Superficial Sensory Radial Nerve

As mentioned previously, the superficial sensory radial nerve runs down the forearm in a cleft between the brachioradialis and extensor carpi radialis longus muscles. After becoming subcutaneous and entering the dorsum of the wrist, this nerve provides sensation to the dorsolateral half of the hand, as well as the proximal two thirds of the second, third, and lateral half of the fourth digits. The more lateral portion of the thumb is also part of this nerve's sensory territory. Opinions differ as to where the most "autonomous" zone for this nerve is located. Some include the anatomical snuff box (between the extensor pollicis longus and brevis tendons), the first dorsal web space, and the area over the distal one half of the second metacarpal bone.

- **There is much variation in sensory territories between the superficial sensory radial nerve and both the dorsal ulnar cutaneous and lateral antebrachial cutaneous nerves. Because of this overlap, isolated lesions to the superficial sensory radial nerve may only yield a small area of sensory loss, which disappears over time. For this reason, the superficial sensory radial nerve is called the *sural nerve of the arm*, and is often harvested for graft repairs or biopsies.**

♦ Clinical Findings and Syndromes

Radial nerve deficits can be profound. Paralysis of wrist and finger extensors is debilitating because without this movement the hand cannot be placed in a functionally useful position. Furthermore, radial sensory deficits to the dorsal hand, although not important for fine finger function, may be misdiagnosed and progress to refractory neuropathic pain syndromes. Triceps palsies are rare because branches to these muscles originate high in the axilla. Even when present, triceps palsies are not too disabling because gravity helps substitute for its action. Following radial nerve injury (traumatic, idiopathic, or iatrogenic), reinnervation is frequently more robust than that seen following either median or ulnar injury, likely because the radial nerve does not innervate any hand intrinsic muscles. Nevertheless, radial nerve controlled finger and thumb extension often does not return. Because these movements are required for proper hand intrinsic function, their permanent paralysis becomes a common indication for tendon transfers.

The Arm

Complete Palsy in the Axilla

Proximal radial nerve palsies are secondary to trauma, pressure palsies, or occasionally from a posteriorly misplaced deltoid injection. Pressure palsies include crutch, Saturday night, and honeymooner's. A high radial palsy (rare) in the axilla can cause both triceps weakness and posterior arm sensory loss, two deficits that distinguish it from more common radial nerve injuries at the spiral groove. Injuries affecting the radial nerve may be differentiated from posterior cord involvement by confirming normal deltoid (axillary off posterior cord) and latissimus dorsi (thoracodorsal off posterior cord) strength. Furthermore, patients with C7 palsies can be distinguished because they usually have numbness in both the volar and dorsal aspects of the third digit (middle finger), with sensory loss not extending proximal to the wrist. Additionally, C7 muscles innervated by the median nerve, including the pronator teres and flexor carpi radialis longus, should also be weak.

A complete radial palsy presents with sensory loss along the posterior arm and forearm, the lower anterolateral arm, as well as the dorsolateral hand. All extensors of the arm are weak. The triceps are weak and the triceps reflex is absent. Forearm flexion may be somewhat weak compared with the normal side, secondary to brachioradialis paralysis. There is a wrist drop from extensor carpi radialis (longus and brevis) and extensor carpi ulnaris weakness. The fingers cannot extend at the knuckle joint. Supination is partially weak, with residual supination performed by the biceps brachii. The wrist and hand appear limp, with the fingers semiflexed and the metacarpal bone of the thumb volar to the palm (**Fig. 3–18**). Distal finger extension is possible secondary to lumbrical function.

♦ **Be aware of certain movements that may mimic true proximal finger extension. When the wrist is flexed, tenodesis causes the fingers to extend. This phenomenon may be exaggerated when sclerosis is present from chronic extensor paralysis. Furthermore, with the fingers partially**

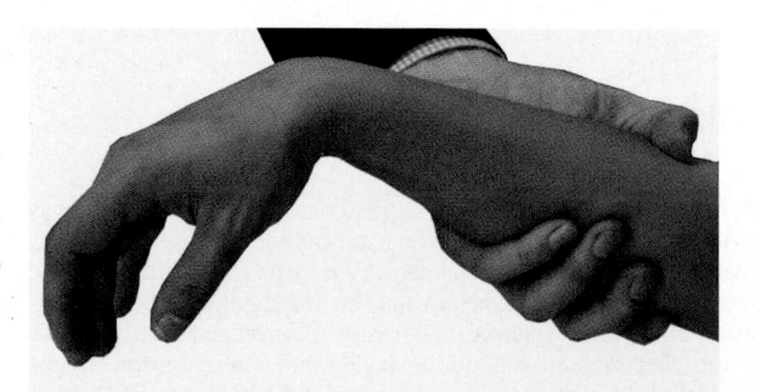

Figure 3–18 Wrist and finger drop secondary to a radial nerve palsy. The wrist and hand appear limp with the fingers semiflexed and the first metacarpal bone (of the thumb) volar to the palm.

flexed, the hand intrinsics may partially extend the knuckle joints. To remove these effects, examine metacarpal joint extension with the wrist held in extension or on a flat surface.

Radial Nerve Damage in the Spiral Groove

The spiral groove is the most common location for traumatic radial nerve palsy. The radial nerve can be directly contused against the humerus, or damaged by a fracture of the midhumeral shaft. It is estimated that approximately 15% of mid-humeral fractures affect the radial nerve. With a humeral fracture, the radial nerve remains tethered where it pierces the lateral intermuscular septum, and because of this immobility, can be transposed between the fractured bone ends (**Fig. 3–19**). A distally misplaced deltoid injection may also damage the radial nerve in this region.

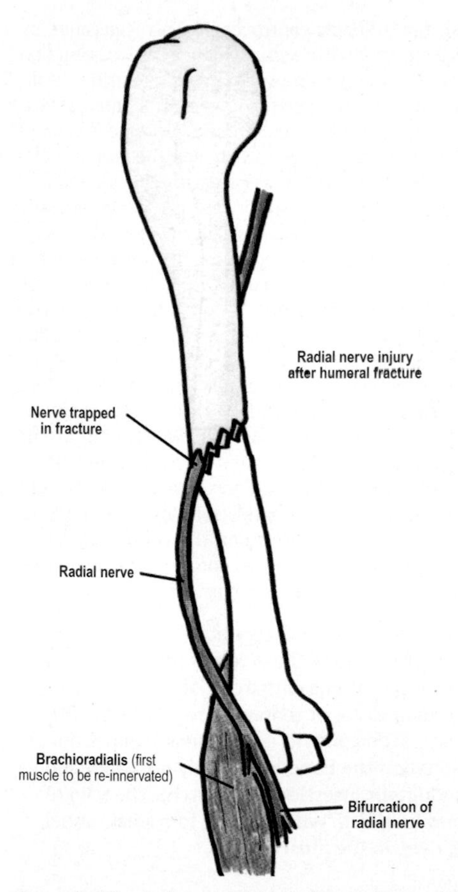

Figure 3–19 Radial nerve injury following humeral fracture. With a humeral fracture, the radial nerve remains tethered where it pierces the lateral intermuscular septum; because of this immobility, it can become pinned between the two ends of fractured bone.

Radial nerve lesions at the spiral groove cause weakness of all muscles distal to the elbow, including the brachioradialis. The triceps are usually spared, as is the triceps reflex. Loss of sensation along the lower lateral arm and posterior forearm usually occurs, whereas the posterior cutaneous nerve to the arm is spared because it does not run in the spiral groove. The brachioradialis is the most proximal muscle to be reinnervated following radial nerve injury at the spiral groove, a process that usually takes 3 to 4 months.

- **In some patients, damage to the radial nerve at the spiral groove may cause mild triceps weakness. This is because supplementary, direct muscular branches to the lateral and medial heads from the radial nerve originate in the spiral groove, where they may be injured.**

The Antecubital Fossa

Radial Tunnel Syndrome

The existence of radial tunnel syndrome remains controversial. This is because, by definition, this syndrome has no objective motor or sensory deficits on examination or electrodiagnostic studies. If these are present, especially finger extension weakness, one must also consider other diagnoses, specifically posterior interosseous nerve compression at the supinator. Anatomically, radial tunnel syndrome is defined as the submuscular path where the radial nerve travels between the lateral intermuscular septum and the supinator. Between these two points, the brachioradialis, extensor carpi radialis longus, and extensor carpi radialis brevis muscles sequentially cover the radial nerve. The extensor carpi radialis brevis actually envelops the nerve, by passing both deep and superficial to it. Some experts propose that irritation of the radial nerve in the radial tunnel can be secondary to an anomalous tendinous ridge on the extensor carpi radialis brevis muscle. Other compression points may include fibrous bands, or irregularities, on the anterior margin of the elbow joint or radial head, or alternatively, a fan of small arterial branches from the recurrent radial artery.

Radial tunnel syndrome and tennis elbow (i.e., lateral epicondylitis) have very similar presentations. Diagnostic criteria for radial tunnel syndrome include (1) being unresponsive to conservative treatment of tennis elbow, (2) pain at the radial tunnel (not the lateral epicondyle) during resisted third digit extension when the elbow is fully extended and the forearm supinated, and (3) nerve tenderness at rest in the radial tunnel. The third digit is believed to instigate the most pain because the extensor carpi radialis brevis inserts on the third metacarpal bone (the extensor carpi radialis longus inserts on the second). Forced supination may also cause pain if the radial tunnel is simultaneously palpated.

- **In contrast, tennis elbow is secondary to forced, repetitive pronation and wrist extension causing inflammation where the extensor muscles attach to the lateral epicondyle. Relief of symptoms with a cortisone injection at the lateral epicondyle is often diagnostic of tennis elbow. Patients with tennis elbow have pain at the lateral epicondyle, not the radial tunnel, and classically have worsened pain when the hand is passively pronated and flexed (putting the effected tendinous insertions on stretch). The pain of tennis elbow is often sharp and localized, whereas that for radial tunnel syndrome is more a dull ache, deep in the muscles.**

Supinator Syndrome

Supinator syndrome is usually a spontaneous palsy of the posterior interosseous nerve secondary to compression or irritation where this nerve enters the supinator muscle. The posterior interosseous nerve passes between the superficial and deep heads of this muscle, analogous to placing your index finger into the front pocket of a pair of jeans. The anterior margin of this "pocket" is termed the arcade of Frohse, and in 30% of the population is very fibrous and thought to predispose to nerve compression (**Fig. 3–20**). Some patients with this syndrome have a history of mild trauma to this region, or alternatively, report repetitive supination movements at work or play.

Patients with supinator syndrome often have pain localized to the supinator muscle, which worsens after a few minutes of forced supination. By history, they have either sudden or progressive finger extension weakness. The supinator muscle itself is classically spared in supinator syndrome because most branches to this muscle occur prior to the nerve entering the muscle. Sensation is normal in the territory of the superficial sensory radial nerve, and the brachioradialis muscle has normal strength. Like radial tunnel syndrome, the existence of supinator syndrome is also somewhat controversial. Some experts believe that many patients diagnosed with this syndrome actually have focal cases of inflammatory neuritis (i.e., Parsonage–Turner syndrome). Therefore, subtle palsies of other upper extremity nerves, as well as any contralateral upper extremity weakness, should be ruled out.

♦ **The healing of a proximal forearm or elbow fracture in misalignment, or with excessive pannus (including from osteomyelitis), may put the posterior interosseous nerve, which is fixed at its entrance into the supinator muscle, under tension. The resultant palsy, termed tardive radial palsy, usually occurs months to years later. This classically occurs after a Monteggia fracture: a proximal ulnar fracture with concurrent posterior dislocation of the radius. Radiographs are diagnostic.**

Patients with rheumatoid arthritis are predisposed to finger extension weakness. They can have synovial thickening at the elbow that compresses

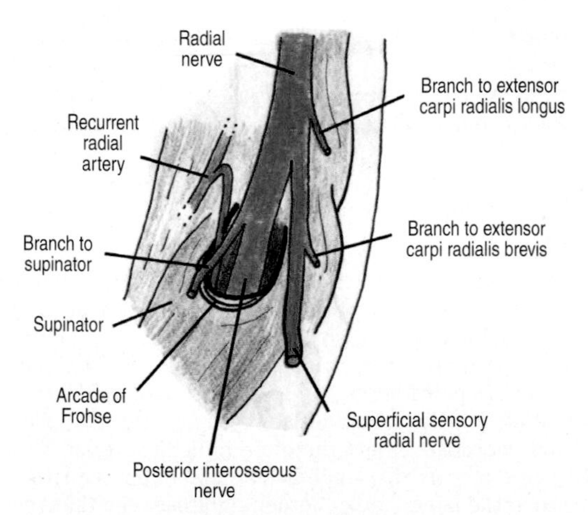

Figure 3–20 Supinator syndrome. The posterior interosseous nerve may be irritated where it enters the supinator muscle. It passes between the superficial and deep heads of this muscle, analogous to placing your index finger into the front pocket of a pair of jeans. The anterior margin of this "pocket" is termed the *arcade of Frohse*, which may be very fibrous and cause nerve compression.

the radial nerve directly or indirectly by elevating the supinator, which places the posterior interosseous nerve on stretch. Rheumatoid arthritis patients can also rupture extensor tendons, which can mimic nerve palsy.

The Forearm

Posterior Interosseous Nerve Palsy

Posterior interosseous nerve palsy can be from trauma, diabetic mononeuropathy, compression at the supinator muscle (supinator syndrome), or from a space-occupying mass, or it can be idiopathic (i.e., Parsonage–Turner syndrome). The most common soft tissue mass compressing the posterior interosseus nerve is a lipoma, followed by nerve sheath tumors, ganglia, and hypertrophic synovium (rheumatoid arthritis). Considering it carries no cutaneous sensory fibers, sensation remains normal when this palsy occurs. However, patients may complain of a dull ache in the proximal forearm extensor muscles, near the radial head.

The motor weakness that occurs in a posterior interosseous palsy has two components: wrist extension weakness in an ulnar direction (radial wrist extension remains normal, mediated by the extensor carpi radialis longus and brevis), and finger extension weakness at the metacarpal-phalangeal joints. Of note, patients do *not* have a wrist drop because the extensor carpi radialis muscles are unaffected. Upon wrist extension, however, the hand deviates in a radial direction because the extensor carpi ulnaris muscle is weak. Isolated posterior interosseous nerve palsy is further confirmed by documenting normal brachioradialis and superficial sensory radial nerve function. Patients with partial posterior interosseous nerve lesions can have variable and progressive weakness in each finger. When weakness begins in only the fourth and fifth digits, a pseudo-ulnar claw hand can be seen. By observation alone, this sign can be easily distinguished because there is no hyperextension at the knuckle joints, as is required for true claw hand.

- ♦ **Supinator and extensor carpi radialis brevis weakness may also occur in a posterior interosseous nerve palsy, depending on each person's specific branching anatomy. Nevertheless, confirming normal brachioradialis and superficial radial sensory nerve function is paramount for making this diagnosis.**

Sensory Radial Nerve Palsy (Wartenberg Syndrome)

Isolated damage to the superficial sensory radial nerve can occur from trauma, tight handcuffs or watches, venipuncture, surgery for de Quervain's tenosynovitis, and occasionally from scissor-like pinching between the brachioradialis and extensor carpi radialis longus tendons. *Wartenberg syndrome* or *cheiralgia paresthetica* are synonymous with superficial sensory radial nerve palsy. Injury to this sensory nerve causes numbness, hyperesthesia, and burning pain on the dorsolateral aspect of the hand. With misdiagnosis and lack of treatment, this pain may become permanent and neuropathic, and therefore difficult to treat. The superficial sensory radial nerve pierces the antebrachial fascia approximately two thirds down the forearm at the lateral radial border, right between the tendons of the brachioradialis and extensor carpi radialis longus (**Fig. 3–21**). With repetitive pronation, the brachioradialis tendon normally closes the space between these two tendons in a scissor-like fashion, potentially irritating the nerve where it emerges from the fascia. In these patients, pain and numbness

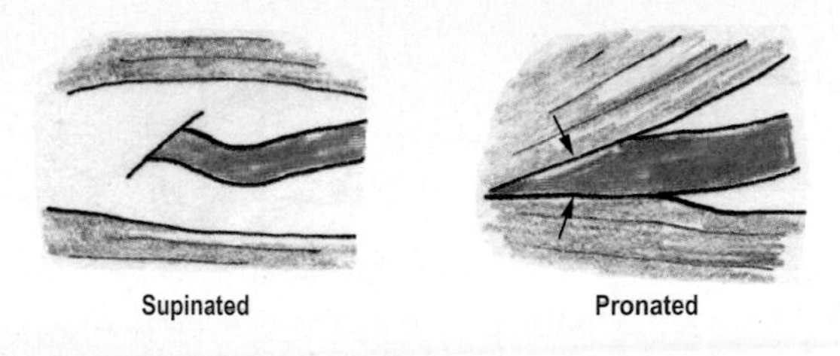

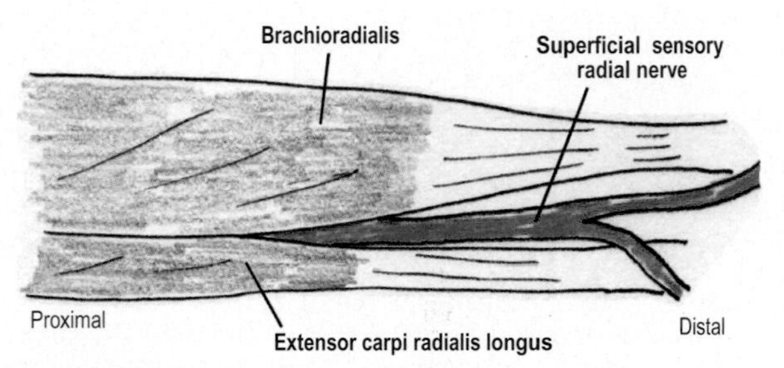

Figure 3–21 Superficial sensory radial nerve entrapment in the distal forearm. With repetitive pronation, the brachioradialis tendon normally closes the space between these two tendons in a scissor-like fashion, potentially irritating the nerve where it emerges from the fascia.

can be exacerbated with simultaneous forced pronation and ulnar wrist deviation, which scissors the tendons together and stretches the nerve, respectively. A Tinel's sign can often be elicited. This diagnosis may be confirmed with electrodiagnostic testing.

- **De Quervain's tenosynovitis, or stenosing tenosynovitis of the first thumb's extensor tendon, may be confused with superficial sensory radial nerve palsy. The *Finkelstein sign* for de Quervain's tenosynovitis occurs if passively bending the hand (as a fist) in an ulnar direction causes pain in the lateral wrist area. A superficial sensory radial nerve palsy may also have a positive Finkelstein sign. These two problems are clinically differentiated by the fact that the nerve palsy more frequently causes sensory loss.**

4

The Diagnostic Anatomy of the Brachial Plexus

Mentioning the phrase "brachial plexus anatomy" is likely to clear a medical school classroom faster than a fire drill. Sure, rout memorization of brachial plexus anatomy out of context can be very frustrating, but this does not have to be the case. For example, when one is familiar with the function of its major, terminal branches (median, ulnar, radial nerves), as well as with that of its spinal nerve input (the C5-T1 nerve roots), learning what comes in between (i.e., the brachial plexus) becomes straightforward. In fact, there is less anatomical detail to absorb than for a single upper extremity nerve.

In this chapter, I will review brachial plexus anatomy with a focus on the student's needs—by systematically discussing the basics, not the minutia. In this chapter, only the most standard anatomy will be presented. Learning variations, despite being both common and important, is best approached after the basics have been mastered.

♦ The Proximal Brachial Plexus

Nerves and Trunks

The brachial plexus is made up of axons from five spinal nerves: C5, C6, C7, C8, and T1. Theses nerves emerge from their respective intervertebral foramina and merge to form the brachial plexus. From each spinal cord segment, multiple ventral (motor) and dorsal (sensory) rootlets exit the spinal cord, coalescing into motor and sensory roots before entering the intervertebral foramen. In the proximal intervertebral foramen, the sensory root enters its spinal ganglion. At the midportion of the intervertebral foramen, the motor and sensory roots merge to form a single spinal nerve. This merger is short-lived, however, because the spinal nerve almost immediately splits into ventral and dorsal rami after exiting the foramen. The dorsal rami of the spinal nerves run posteriorly to innervate paraspinal muscles and skin; the ventral rami form the brachial plexus.

As the spinal nerves pass through the intervertebral foramen, their enveloping dura gradually turns into epineurium. The primary site of adherence, or stabilization, of these spinal nerves is located just outside the foramen, where the inferior aspect of the nerve is attached to a depression in the transverse process. This is the only bony attachment of the brachial plexus, and serves to protect the weak intradural rootlets from traction injury that may cause traumatic avulsion. This attachment is well developed for C5, C6, and C7, but is weak or absent for C8 and T1, making these latter two nerves more susceptible to avulsion injury.

Immediately on formation, the ventral rami, which are destined for the brachial plexus, communicate with the sympathetic ganglia. This connection with the sympathetic nervous system includes both gray and white rami. More proximally, the gray ramus carries postsynaptic fibers from the sympathetic ganglia to the spinal nerve; they are destined for sweat glands and vasoconstrictors. The slightly more distal white ramus carries preganglionic information from the spinal cord to the sympathetic ganglia.

Of importance, the sympathetic fibers destined for the face via the trigeminal nerve originate from the upper thoracic spinal cord, travel through the T1 and T2 spinal nerves, and pass via the white rami into the paravertebral ganglia. These sympathetic axons pass cranially, ultimately terminating in the superior cervical ganglion. Postsynaptic sympathetic axons exit this ganglion and enter the head upon the internal carotid artery, only to be subsequently transferred to the trigeminal nerve in the cavernous sinus. Following the branches of the trigeminal nerve, these axons mediate facial sweating, pupillary dilatation, and contraction of tarsal muscles and Mueller's muscle. Therefore, with damage to the T1 and/or T2 spinal nerves, one can have *Horner's syndrome*: anhidrosis (lack of sweating), miosis (lack of pupillary dilatation), ptosis (tarsal muscle weakness), and enophthalmus (palsy of Mueller's muscle). The presence of a Horner's syndrome is a sign of very proximal injury to the brachial plexus.

The two upper roots, C5 and C6, merge to become the upper trunk. The lower two roots, C8 and T1, travel a bit cranially over the first rib to form the lower trunk. This leaves the C7 root to create the middle trunk. These three trunks (upper, middle, and lower), once formed, travel distal toward the clavicle (**Fig. 4–1**). The middle and lower trunks, as well as the C8 and T1 spinal nerves, usually do not have any branches of clinical significance. Excluding variations, the only branches from the proximal brachial plexus originate from the C5, C6, and C7 spinal nerves, as well as the upper trunk.

From the spine to the clavicle, the spinal nerves and trunks run sandwiched between the anterior and middle scalene muscles (the *scalenes*). The only

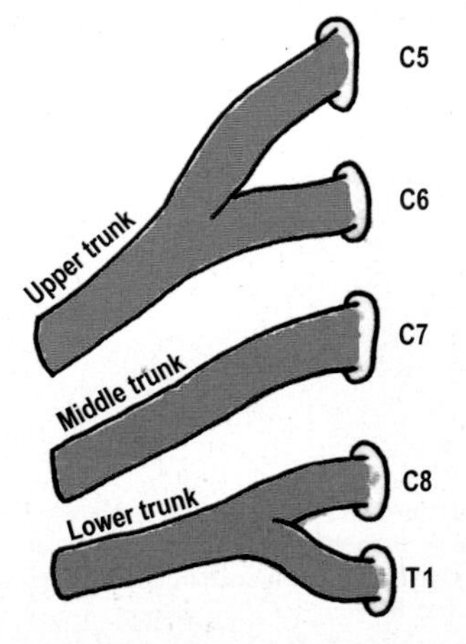

Figure 4–1 Proximal brachial plexus: spinal nerves to trunks without branches. The two upper roots, C5 and C6, merge to become the upper trunk, while the lower two roots, C8 and T1, travel a bit cranially over the first rib to form the lower trunk. That leaves only the C7 root to create the middle trunk.

components of the supraclavicular brachial plexus not completely covered by these two muscles are C5, C6, and a proximal segment of the upper trunk. The point where C5 and C6 merge to create the upper trunk, is called *Erb's point*. C8 and T1 start below the scalenes, but initially rise cranially to be flanked by them.

- **Prior to entering the brachial plexus, the spinal nerves are commonly referred to as roots. Although this nomenclature is not correct, it is commonly used. Occasionally, either C4 or T2 may contribute to the brachial plexus. When there is C4 contribution and a small T1 input, the brachial plexus is considered prefixed. In contrast, when there is minor C5 spinal nerve input with a definite T2 contribution, the plexus is called postfixed.**

The Spinal Nerve Branches

Three nerves receive fibers from the C5 nerve root: the phrenic nerve to the diaphragm, long thoracic nerve to the serratus anterior, and the dorsal scapular nerve to the rhomboid muscles. C6 and C7 also provide fibers to the long thoracic nerve (**Fig. 4–2**). As mentioned, no important branches usually arise from the C8 and T1 spinal nerves.

The Phrenic Nerve

The C5 spinal nerve provides input to the phrenic nerve. The phrenic nerve is made up of motor fibers from C3, C4, and C5; hence, the phrase "C3, 4, and 5

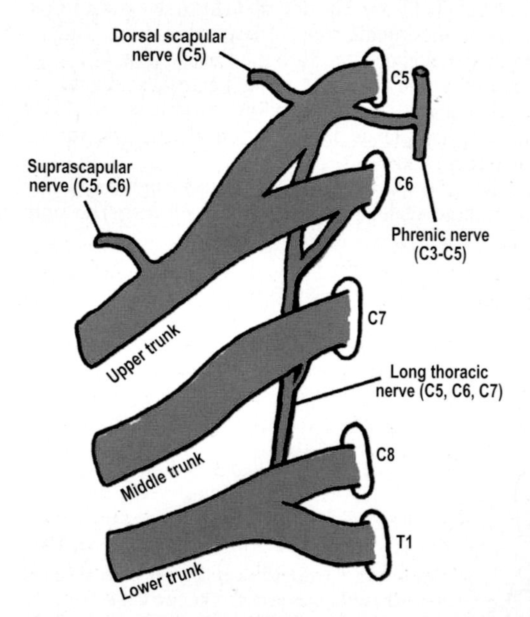

Figure 4–2 Proximal brachial plexus: spinal nerves to trunks with branches. Three branches receive a contribution from the C5 nerve root: the phrenic, long thoracic, and dorsal scapular. C6 and C7 also contribute to the long thoracic nerve. One important branch originates from the upper trunk: the suprascapular nerve.

keeps a man alive." After being formed, the phrenic nerve runs distally on the superficial aspect of the anterior scalene muscle, laterally to medially (it is the only nerve that runs laterally to medially in the posterior triangle). Along with the anterior scalene, the phrenic nerve passes between the subclavian artery located posteriorly and the subclavian vein anteriorly, to enter the thorax. Each phrenic nerve innervates one *hemidiaphragm*. Depending on the amount of C5 input to the phrenic nerve, a very proximal lesion to the C5 nerve root may cause an ipsilaterally elevated and paralyzed diaphragm. This may be diagnosed by comparing the percussion of both lungs during inspiration. A radiograph or ultrasound will also confirm this type of paralysis.

Phrenic nerve damage may occur during open-heart surgery; it is associated with the use of ice slush to cool the heart. When this occurs postoperatively, it is thought to be a cause of respirator dependence, especially when bilateral palsies are present.

The Long Thoracic Nerve

Another branch from the proximal brachial plexus is the long thoracic nerve, having intraforaminal contributions from C5, C6, and C7. The long thoracic nerve forms dorsal to the spinal nerves, travels behind the proximal brachial plexus caudally between the anterior and middle scalenes, over the posterolateral portion of the first rib, eventually innervating the *serratus anterior* muscle. The serratus anterior pulls the scapula away from the midline and forward around the thorax (scapular abduction). It also rotates the scapular upward. Most importantly, however, this muscle fixes and stabilizes the scapula so that muscles originating from it can function properly.

Injury to the long thoracic nerve causes winging of the scapula. At rest, there may be prominence of the scapula's inferomedial edge, with medial displacement and downward rotation. Winging is classically worsened when the patient pushes forward against resistance with the elbow fully extended and the shoulder girdle protracted forward (anterior) (**Fig. 4–3**). This latter finding is the hallmark of a long thoracic palsy.

To test this muscle, instruct the patient to reach for a point on the wall in front of him or her, and then apply resistance at the hand or wrist while stabilizing the thorax with the other hand. A common mistake is to not have the patient displace the shoulder girdle forward enough because without doing so, scapular winging from trapezius or rhomboid weakness may be misdiagnosed as a long thoracic palsy. Of note, weakness of any of these three muscles can cause winging when the arm is pushed against resistance across the chest with the arm bent.

- **The C7 spinal nerve variably provides a branch to the long thoracic nerve. Although weakness itself of the serratus anterior often causes a dull ache in the shoulder region, if the pain is acute and severe, then one should consider acute brachial neuritis as the etiology.**

The Dorsal Scapular Nerve

Another branch from the C5 spinal root is the dorsal scapular nerve. This nerve innervates both the major and minor *rhomboid muscles* (the rhomboids). The rhomboids connect the medial edge of the scapula to the spinal column. When contracted, the rhomboids pull the scapula toward the midline (scapular adduction) and superiorly (scapular downward rotation)—the opposite direction to that of the serratus anterior muscle. The dorsal scapular nerve passes dorsally perforating the middle scalene. It then travels along the undersurface of the levator scapulae down to the rhomboids. With chronic denervation of the rhomboids,

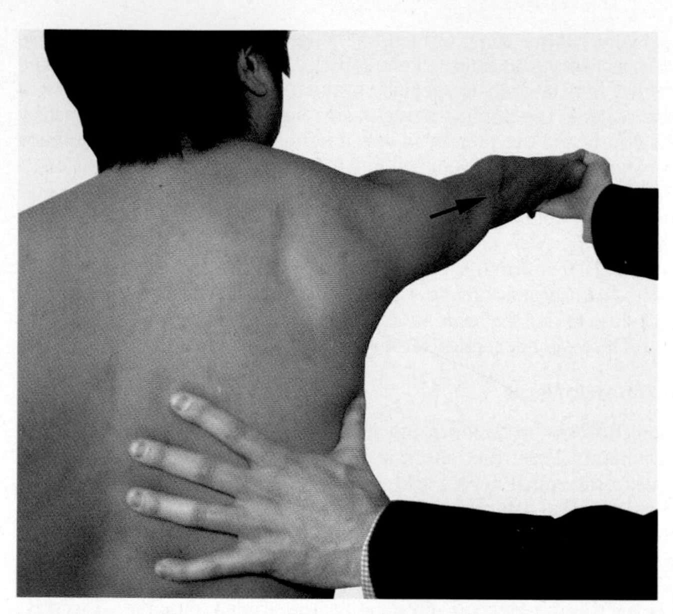

Figure 4–3 Serratus anterior (C5, C6, C7) assessment: Instruct the patient to reach for a point on the wall in front of him or her, and then apply resistance at the wrist while stabilizing the thorax with your other hand. A common mistake is to not have the patient displace the shoulder girdle forward enough (i.e., enough shoulder protraction) because without doing so, scapular winging from trapezius or rhomboid weakness may be misdiagnosed as a long thoracic palsy.

interscapular wasting is evident. With rhomboid weakness, there may be mild scapular winging at rest, especially at the inferomedial edge. The scapula may also be laterally displaced and upwardly rotated. To test the rhomboids have the patient place the palm on his or her lower back facing outward. Instruct the patient to push the palm away from the lower back as you apply resistance to the hand as well as to the arm (apply resistance in an anterolateral direction around the thorax) **(Fig. 4–4)**. Observe and palpate the rhomboids during this maneuver. Concurrent damage to the proximal brachial plexus is often present; therefore, the forearm may need to be supported. An alternate method to examine the rhomboids is to have the patient bring the shoulders and scapulae together posteriorly. In this position, the contracted rhomboids can be palpated between the medial aspects of the scapulae.

- **The dorsal scapular nerve can provide partial innervation to the levator scapula as it passes underneath this muscle.**

The Truncal Branches

There is only one branch of significance from the brachial plexus trunks: the suprascapular nerve. This nerve originates from the distal, superior aspect of the upper trunk, just above the clavicle. In summary, therefore, all the proximal brachial plexus branches come from the C5, C6, and C7 spinal nerves, or the upper trunk, with C5 input being present in all of them (**Fig. 4–2**).

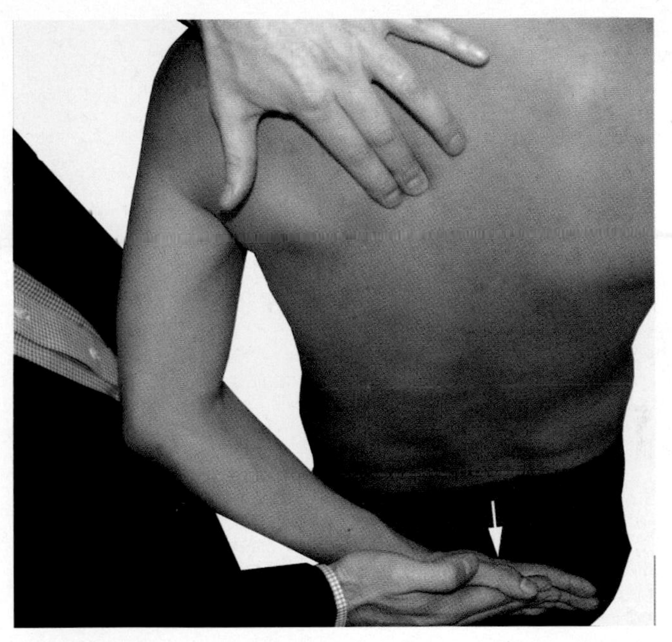

Figure 4–4 Major and minor rhomboids (C5) assessment: Have the patient place the palm facing outward on his or her lower back. Instruct the patient to push the palm away from the lower back as you apply resistance to the hand as well as to the arm (the arm is pushed anterior and lateral around the thorax). Instruct the patient to lead with the hand, not the elbow.

The Suprascapular Nerve

The *suprascapular nerve* (C5, C6) descends posteriorly and distally along the superior portion of the upper trunk, then between the inferior belly of the omohyoid and the trapezius muscle toward the suprascapular notch. The suprascapular nerve's convergence with the omohyoid muscle at the scapula confirms its identity. The suprascapular artery and vein traverse the brachial plexus just superior and deep to the clavicle, joining the suprascapular nerve as it approaches the suprascapular notch. The suprascapular nerve passes through the notch and under the superior scapular ligament; the artery and vein pass over this ligament (**Fig. 4–5**). The nerve and vessels join again as they pass around the lateral edge of the scapular spine through the spinoglenoid fossa. Here, all components of the neurovascular bundle pass under the inferior scapular ligament. The suprascapular nerve innervates the *supraspinatus* and *infraspinatus* muscles. The supraspinatus attaches to the superior aspect of the humeral head and mediates the initial 20 to 30 degrees of arm abduction. The infraspinatus attaches to the posterior aspect of the humeral head and is the primary external rotator of the arm. Test the supraspinatus muscle by having the patient abduct a straight arm from his or her side against resistance (**Fig. 4–6**). To test the infraspinatus muscle, instruct the patient to flex the forearm to 90 degrees. Then stabilize the elbow against the side of the patient, and ask him or her to rotate the arm externally against resistance,

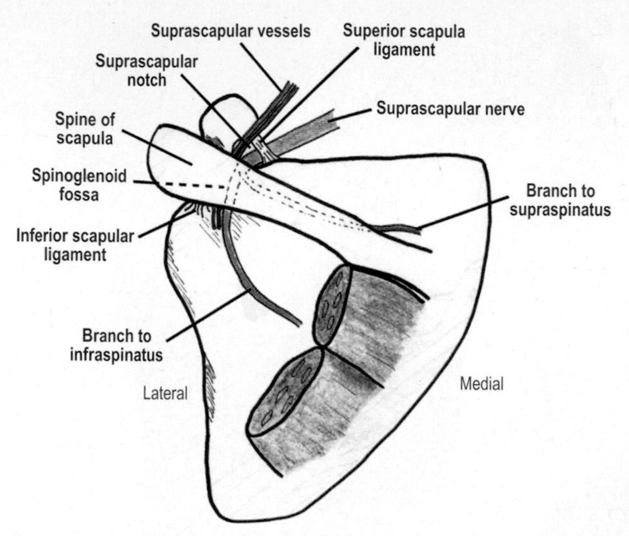

Figure 4–5 Suprascapular anatomy. The suprascapular nerve passes under the superior scapular ligament; the artery and vein pass over this ligament. This neurovascular bundle then passes around the lateral edge of the scapular spine through the spinoglenoid fossa. Here both the vessels and nerve pass under the inferior scapular ligament.

like a tennis swing (**Fig. 4–7**). Contraction of these two muscles can be observed and palpated during testing. With chronic denervation, atrophy above (supraspinatus) or below (infraspinatus) the scapular spine is readily appreciated.

Acute suprascapular palsies are usually secondary to trauma (abrupt shoulder distraction or scapular fractures); therefore, for gradual-onset palsies one should consider ganglion cysts or idiopathic entrapment at the suprascapular

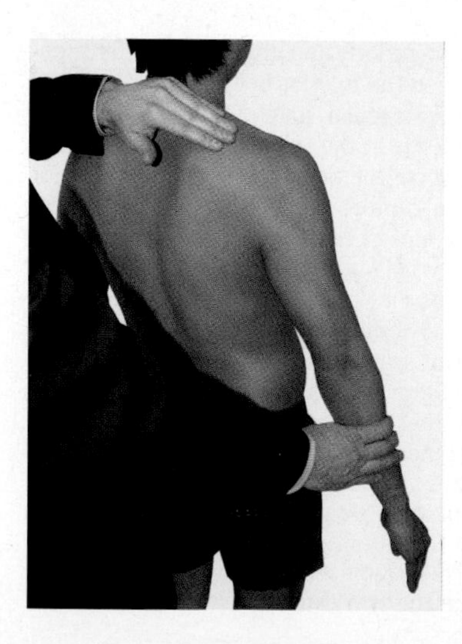

Figure 4–6 Supraspinatus (C5, C6) assessment: Test the supraspinatus muscle by having the patient abduct a straight arm from his or her side against resistance.

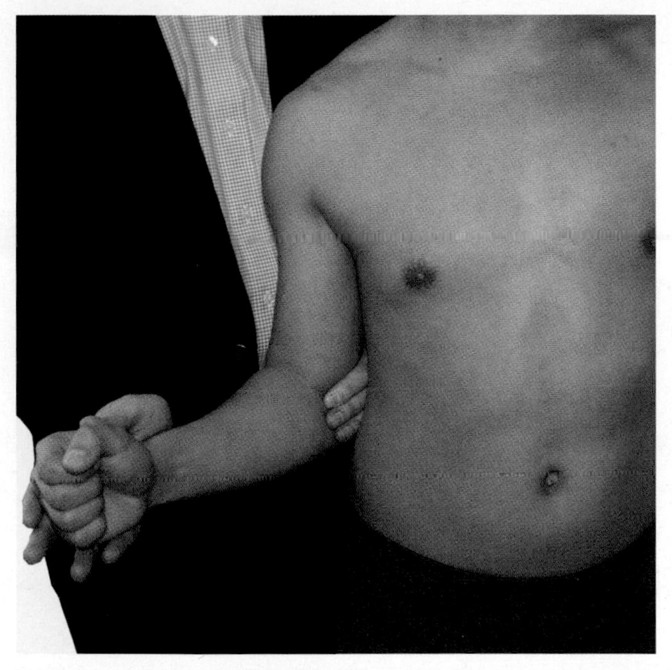

Figure 4–7 Infraspinatus (C5, C6) assessment: Test the infraspinatus muscle by instructing the patient to flex the forearm to 90 degrees. Then stabilize the elbow against the side of the patient, and ask him or her to rotate the arm externally against resistance, like a tennis swing. (The teres minor also externally rotates the arm.)

notch. If there is a great deal of shoulder pain that improves as muscle weakness appears, then acute brachial neuritis is likely. For entrapment cases, narrowing or callus involving the suprascapular notch may be seen on properly directed radiographs.

♦ **The small, often forgotten, subclavius nerve to the subclavius muscle also originates from the upper trunk. This muscle, however, cannot be tested clinically or electrophysiologically; therefore, it is unimportant.**

♦ The Distal Brachial Plexus

Major Branches from the Cords

The distal portion of the brachial plexus is composed of cords, which are named according to their relationship to the axillary artery deep to the pectoralis minor muscle (lateral, medial, posterior)(**Fig. 4–8**). The cords are intimately associated with the axillary artery and vein in this region. As the brachial plexus cords pass further distal to the pectoralis minor, their anatomical relationship to this artery changes—they are no longer lateral, medial, and posterior.

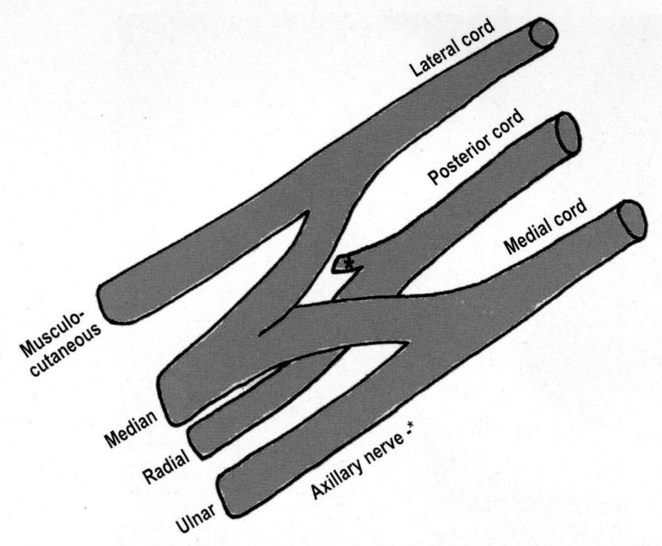

Figure 4–8 Distal brachial plexus cords and terminal branches. The distal portion of the brachial plexus is composed of cords, which are named according to their relationship to the axillary artery deep to the pectoralis minor (lateral, medial, posterior).

The major, terminal branches of the brachial plexus have been discussed in previous chapters (median, ulnar, and radial nerves). The median nerve is not a continuation of any cord per se, but is created from a lateral contribution from the lateral cord (mostly sensory), as well as a medial contribution from the medial cord (mostly motor to hand intrinsics). Both of these contributions pass superficial to the axillary artery and form the median nerve on its anterior surface. After giving these contributions, the remaining portion of the medial cord continues into the arm as the ulnar nerve; the remaining portion of the lateral cord continues as the musculocutaneous nerve. This anatomical arrangement resembles an M over the axillary artery, with the center leg being the median nerve, the lateral leg the musculocutaneous nerve, and the medial leg the ulnar nerve. The posterior cord runs deep to the axillary artery. In the axilla, the posterior cord remains deep between the axillary artery and vein, with the axillary nerve branching off, prior to it continuing as the radial nerve into the arm. The musculocutaneous and axillary nerves will be discussed further at this point.

The Musculocutaneous Nerve

The *musculocutaneous nerve* (C5, C6) is the distal continuation of the lateral cord containing fibers from the upper trunk (**Fig. 4–9**). In the axilla, the musculocutaneous nerve travels distal, and somewhat lateral, to pierce the *coracobrachialis* muscle, which it innervates. The coracobrachialis muscle assists the anterior deltoid in flexing the arm (forward in front of the body). It also stabilizes the humerus during forearm flexion. The coracobrachialis cannot be isolated or palpated, and therefore, is not examined clinically. After passing through, and then deep to this muscle, the musculocutaneous nerve continues on the superficial surface of the *brachialis* muscle deep to the lateral border of the *biceps*

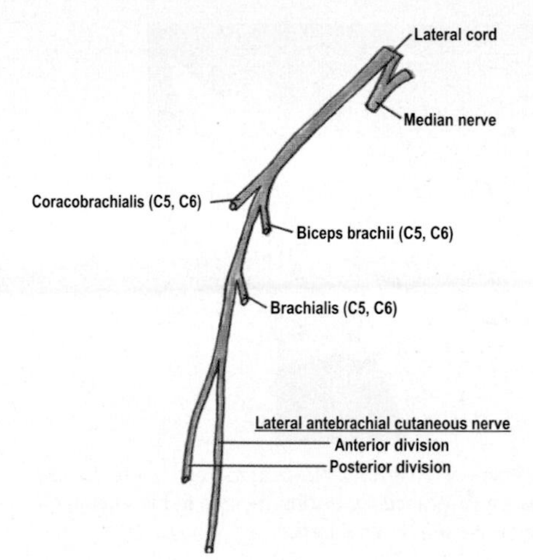

Figure 4–9 Motor innervation of the musculocutaneous nerve.

brachii. These two muscles are also innervated via multiple branches off the musculocutaneous nerve. Distally, the musculocutaneous nerve enters the antecubital fossa where it pierces the superficial fascia just lateral to the biceps tendon, entering the subcutaneous space as the *lateral antebrachial cutaneous nerve.* The territory of this sensory nerve includes, as the name implies, the lateral half of the forearm (**Fig. 4–10**). The lateral antebrachial cutaneous nerve has an anterior and posterior division. The biceps brachii, with the assistance of the brachialis and brachioradialis, flexes the forearm. The biceps brachii is also a strong supinator of the forearm when the elbow is flexed. To test the biceps brachii and brachialis, have the patient flex a fully supinated arm against resistance

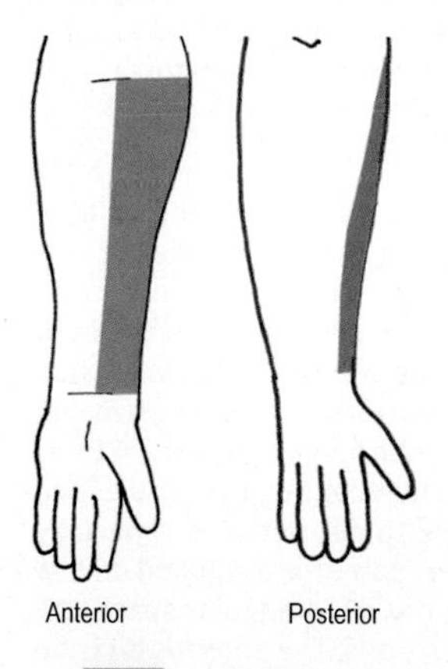

Figure 4–10 Musculocutaneous nerve sensory territory. The territory of the lateral antebrachial cutaneous nerve includes, as the name implies, the lateral one half of the forearm.

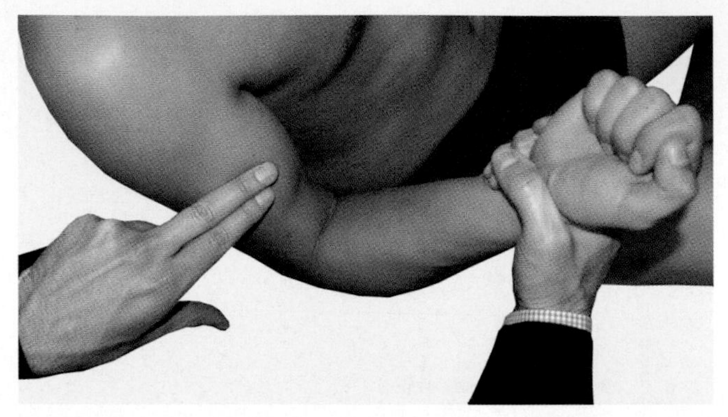

Figure 4–11 Biceps brachii (C5, C6) assessment: To test the biceps brachii and brachialis, have the patient flex a fully supinated arm against resistance. By testing the arm in full supination, contribution from the brachioradialis (radial nerve) is minimized.

(**Fig. 4–11**). By testing the arm in full supination, the contribution from the brachioradialis is minimized.

Isolated musculocutaneous palsies are rare, but can occur occasionally following trauma or shoulder dislocation. These patients would present with numbness in their anterolateral forearm and with forearm flexion weakness. These findings need to be clinically differentiated from a biceps tendon rupture, as well as from a C6 radiculopathy. Following tendon rupture, the biceps still contracts and can be felt rolling up the arm. A C6 radiculopathy can also be differentiated not only because of the radicular pain, but also because of possible weakness in other, non-musculocutaneous innervated, C6 muscles, including the brachioradialis and latissimus dorsi. Furthermore, C6 radiculopathies usually cause numbness confined to the thumb and index finger, whereas the sensory coverage of the lateral antebrachial cutaneous nerve stops at the wrist. Focal damage to the lateral antebrachial cutaneous nerve can be from venipuncture in the antecubital fossa.

The Axillary Nerve

The *axillary nerve* (C5, C6) arises from the posterior cord deep to the axillary artery. A branch off the axillary artery, the posterior humeral circumflex artery, joins the axillary nerve, passing inferiorly and medially to it. This neurovascular bundle passes briefly upon the subscapularis muscle toward the surgical neck of the humerus. It then passes through the *quadrangular, or quadrilateral, space*, which is bordered superiorly by the teres minor, inferiorly by the teres major, laterally by the neck of the humerus, and medially by the long head of the triceps (**Fig. 4–12**). The axillary nerve is relatively fixed at the quadrangular space, and analogous to the suprascapular nerve in the suprascapular notch, is especially vulnerable to stretch injury when blunt or traction forces are applied to the brachial plexus. Immediately after passing through the quadrangular space, the axillary nerve divides into anterior and posterior divisions. The anterior division curves anteriorly and somewhat superiorly under the *deltoid muscle*, which it innervates. The posterior division gives an immediate branch to the *teres minor* after passing through the quadrangular space (**Fig. 4–13**). The posterior division then pierces the brachial fascia distal and posterior to the deltoid's insertion into

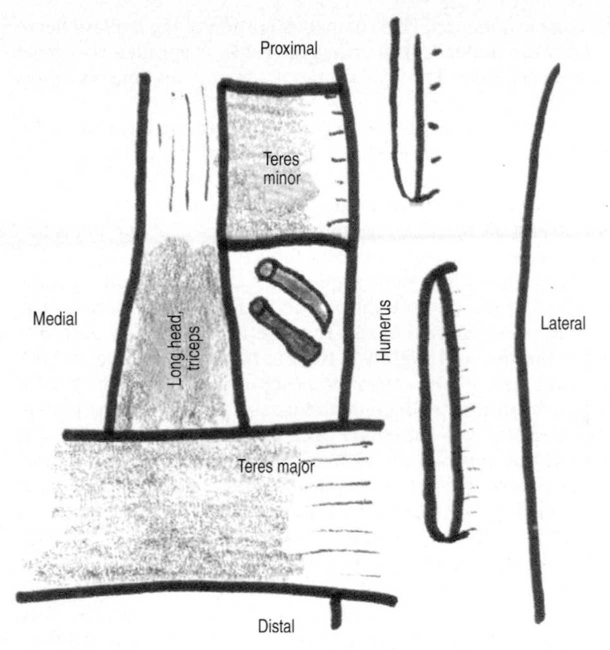

Figure 4–12 Borders of the quadrangular space, ventral perspective. The axillary nerve passes through the quadrangular space, which is bordered superiorly by the teres minor, inferiorly by the teres major, laterally by the neck of the humerus, and medially by the long head of the triceps.

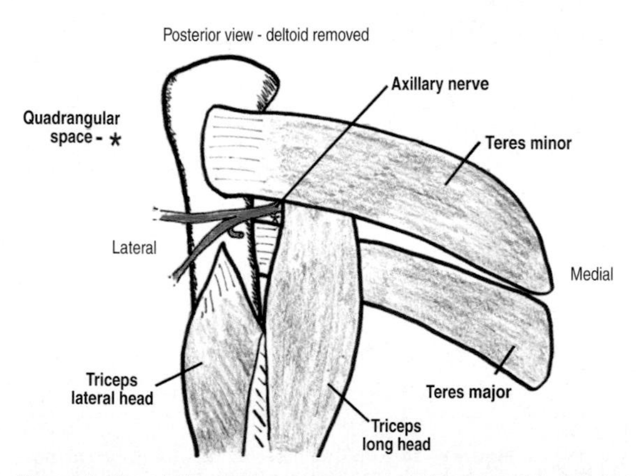

Figure 4–13 Axillary nerve anatomy, posterior view with deltoid removed. Immediately after passing through the quadrangular space, the axillary nerve divides into an anterior and posterior division. The anterior division curves anteriorly and somewhat superiorly under the deltoid muscle, which it innervates. The posterior division gives an immediate branch to the teres minor after passing through the quadrangular space, and then becomes subcutaneous by piercing the brachial fascia.

the humerus to become cutaneous. This cutaneous portion of the axillary nerve carries sensation from the upper lateral arm (**Fig. 4–14**); it is called the *upper lateral brachial cutaneous nerve*. The axillary nerve also carries sensory fibers from the shoulder joint.

The teres minor assists the infraspinatus in externally rotating the arm. It also weakly assists the teres major in adducting a straight arm. It is not possible to test the teres minor in complete isolation, but one may observe and palpate its contraction if the patient is thin. The deltoid is the prime abductor of the arm, especially between 30 and 90 degrees. The initial 30 degrees of abduction is primarily controlled by the supraspinatus, whereas abduction above 90 degrees has an important trapezial component, which rotates the shoulder girdle upward. Test the deltoid by having the patient abduct the arm against resistance (**Fig. 4–15**). The deltoid has three separate heads: the anterior, lateral, and posterior. Abducting the arm to the side and slightly in front of the body tests the anterior and lateral heads of the deltoid. To assess the posterior head, have the patient place a straightened arm almost 90 degrees abducted, and then ask the patient to move the arm posteriorly and superiorly against resistance (**Fig. 4–16**). The absence of posterior deltoid contraction can help confirm an axillary palsy, especially in those patients with a powerful supraspinatus muscle that alone can abduct the arm to 90 degrees. Arm flexion (in front of the body) is mediated by the anterior deltoid. Although the initial 60 degrees of arm flexion is mostly anterior deltoid, the serratus anterior assists the deltoid during flexion above 60 degrees.

The axillary nerve is usually injured in isolation by shoulder trauma, including shoulder dislocations or humeral fractures. For patients with suspected axillary neuropathy following shoulder trauma, one should always exclude partial damage to the posterior division of the brachial plexus as an alternate diagnosis.

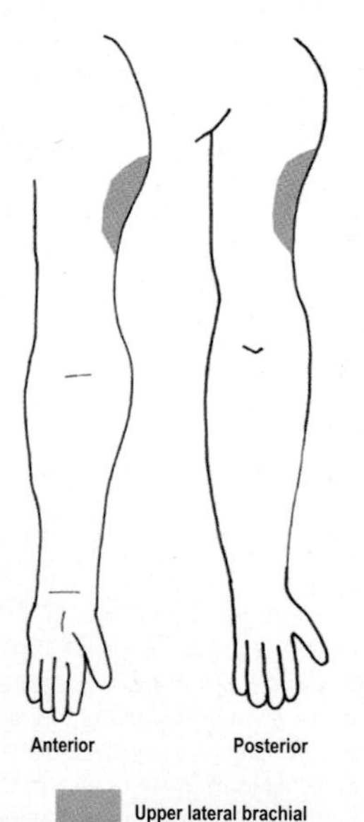

Figure 4–14 Axillary nerve sensory territory. The posterior division of the axillary nerve ends by piercing the brachial fascia distal and posterior to the deltoid's insertion into the humerus. This cutaneous extension of the axillary nerve carries sensation from the upper lateral arm, and is called the *upper lateral brachial cutaneous nerve*.

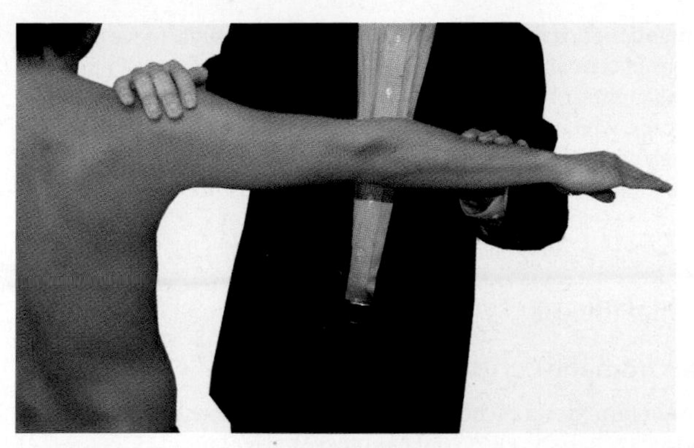

Figure 4–15 Deltoid (C5, C6) assessment: Test the deltoid by having the patient abduct the arm against resistance. The deltoid has three separate heads: anterior, lateral, and posterior. Abducting the arm to the side, and slightly in front of the body tests the anterior and lateral heads of the deltoid. The deltoid controls abduction between 30 and 90 degrees.

By examining the latissimus dorsi (the thoracodorsal nerve), as well as all the muscles innervated by the radial nerve, posterior cord involvement can be excluded. The axillary nerve may be compressed at the quadrangular space, which is known as the *quadrangular space syndrome*. The etiology of this entrapment is uncertain.

- **Sensory loss on the upper lateral arm is usually only temporary, even with complete axillary palsies. This is because following injury the descending cervical plexus branches to supply sensation to this area. Even with complete deltoid paralysis, the patient may use other upper-extremity muscles to abduct the arm, thereby mimicking deltoid**

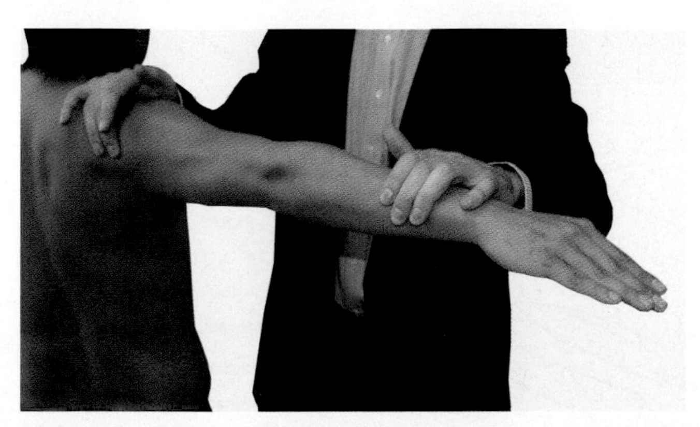

Figure 4–16 Posterior deltoid (C5, C6) assessment: To assess the posterior deltoid, have the patient place a straightened arm almost 90 degrees abducted, and then ask him or her to move the arm posteriorly and superiorly against resistance. Contraction of the posterior head can be observed and palpated.

function. As mentioned, a well-developed supraspinatus can achieve more than 30 degrees of arm abduction. The external rotators of the arm may also weakly abduct the arm. In addition, both the coracobrachialis and long head of the triceps, which connect the scapula to the humerus and olecranon, respectively, can substitute for deltoid function by lifting the arm. Therefore, palpating the deltoid during muscle testing is important.

♦ Distal Brachial Plexus

Minor Branches from the Cords

Aside from the major terminal branches described in the previous section (musculocutaneous and axillary nerves), each cord has other smaller branches (**Fig. 4–17**). The lateral cord gives one minor branch, the lateral pectoral nerve to the pectoralis major. The medial cord gives three minor branches, a medial pectoral nerve to both the pectoralis minor and major, and two cutaneous branches: the medial brachial and antebrachial cutaneous nerves. The posterior cord also has three small branches: It has two subscapular nerves, the upper subscapular to the subscapularis and the lower subscapular to the subscapularis and teres major, as well as a third branch called the thoracodorsal nerve, which innervates the latissimus dorsi. Damage to any of these nerves helps localize a lesion to the cord level.

The Lateral Cord

The *lateral pectoral nerve* (C5, C6) branches from the proximal lateral cord, travels over the brachial plexus and axillary artery, pierces the clavipectoral fascia (which separates the pectoralis major from all other deep structures, including the pectoralis minor), and then fans out to innervate the *pectoralis major* from below. The lateral pectoral nerve concentrates its innervation upon the clavicular head of the pectoralis major. When this branch passes over the plexus, there is a reliable

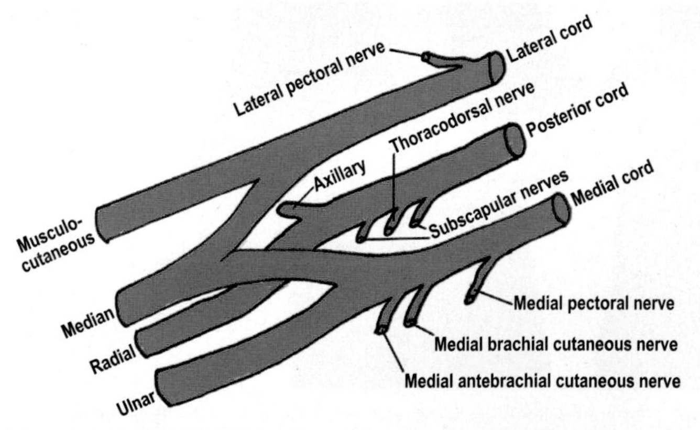

Figure 4–17 Distal brachial plexus and branches. Aside from the major terminal branches, each cord has other smaller branches: The lateral cord has one, and both the medial and posterior cords have three.

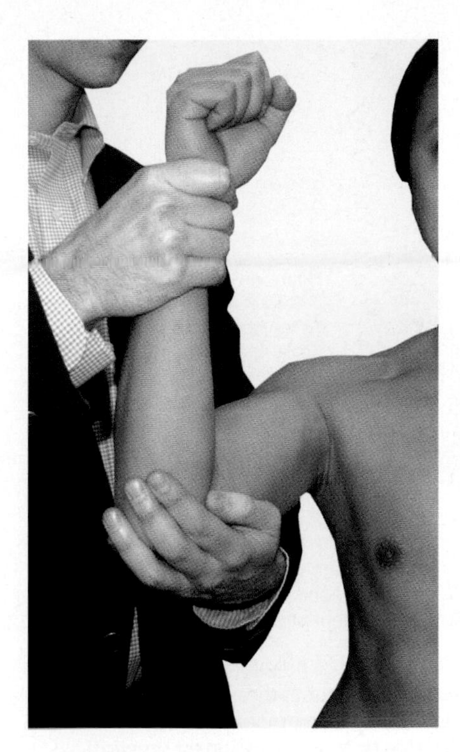

Figure 4–18 Clavicular head of the pectoralis major (C5, C6) assessment: To test the clavicular head of the pectoralis major, start by having the patient abduct the arm 90 degrees with the forearm in flexion and palm facing forward. Then, against resistance at the medial elbow, instruct the patient to swing his or her arm anterior toward the midline (across the chest).

connection, or temporary merger, with the medial pectoral nerve, which as the name implies, comes from the medial cord. The pectoralis major is a strong adductor and internal rotator of the arm. To test the clavicular head of the pectoralis major, and therefore the lateral pectoral nerve, have the patient abduct the arm 90 degrees with the forearm flexed and palm facing forward (**Fig. 4–18**). Then, against resistance at the medial elbow, have the patient swing his or her arm toward midline. The lateral pectoral nerve is the only minor branch from the lateral cord.

The Medial Cord

There are three minor branches from the medial trunk: the more proximal medial pectoral nerve, and the more distal medial brachial and antebrachial cutaneous nerves. The *medial pectoral nerve* (C6-T1) innervates the *pectoralis minor*, which it passes through, and then pierces the clavipectoral fascia to innervate the sternal head of the *pectoralis major*. As mentioned, this nerve almost always communicates with the lateral pectoral nerve. To test the sternal head of the pectoralis major, the patient should begin with the forearm flexed 90 degrees and the arm abducted approximately 30 degrees. Instruct the patient to adduct the arm against resistance placed at the medial elbow (**Fig. 4–19**). The pectoralis minor cannot be adequately isolated from the pectoralis major, and is therefore not assessed clinically.

Just prior to formation of the ulnar nerve, the medial cord gives off two branches: the *medial brachial cutaneous nerve* and the *medial antebrachial cutaneous nerve*. Both of these nerves were discussed in the ulnar nerve chapter because they are

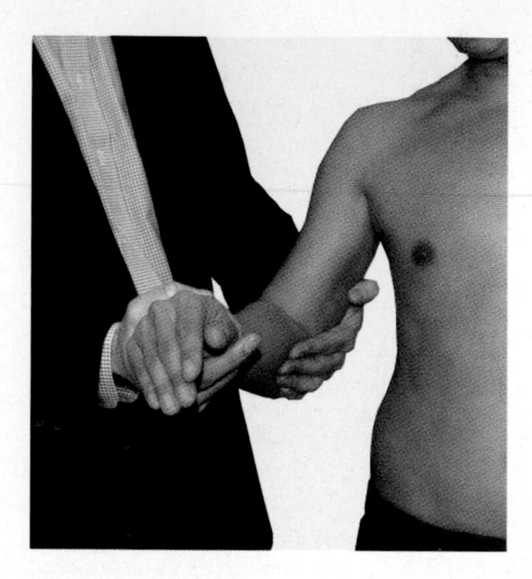

Figure 4–19 Sternal head of the pectoralis major (C6-T1) assessment: To test the sternal head of the pectoralis major, the patient begins with the forearm flexed 90 degrees and the arm abducted approximately 30 degrees. Then instruct the patient to adduct the arm against resistance applied to the medial elbow.

more readily understood in that context. In summary, sensory loss on the medial one half of the arm (medial brachial cutaneous) and forearm (medial antebrachial cutaneous) should be used to confirm involvement of the medial cord.

- **The medial arm is part of the T2 dermatome. Therefore, the medial antebrachial cutaneous nerve returns sensory impulses through the medial cord and lower trunk to the T2 spinal nerve. The presence of T2 axons in the brachial plexus has been excluded thus far from discussion for simplicity.**

Posterior Cord

Like the medial cord, the posterior cord also has three minor branches. The muscles they innervate are easy to remember because they are the same three muscles upon which the radial nerve (terminal continuation of the posterior cord) passes superficial to when exiting the axilla: the subscapularis, latissimus dorsi, and teres major. All three of these branches hang down like icicles from the posterior cord over the surface of the subscapularis muscle.

The first and last minor branches from the posterior cord are aptly named the *upper and lower subscapular nerves* (C5, C6). The upper subscapular nerve is not very long and enters the *subscapularis muscle* to innervate it. The subscapularis muscle, along with the teres major (and latissimus dorsi and pectoralis major), internally rotates the arm. The subscapularis muscle cannot be completely isolated, but one can test internal arm rotation as a composite test (**Fig. 4–20**). The lower subscapular nerve innervates the lower half of the subscapularis muscle, as well as the teres major. The teres major, along with the latissimus dorsi and pectoralis major, are the main arm adductors. To test the teres major, begin with a straightened arm abducted horizontally with the palm down. Instruct the patient to adduct the extended arm against resistance while you inspect the teres major (**Fig. 4–21**). The third branch from the posterior cord is the *thoracodorsal nerve*, which arises between the upper and lower subscapular nerves. The thoracodorsal nerve innervates the latissimus dorsi muscle. To assess the latissimus dorsi, the patient should adduct the arm when the forearm is flexed 90 degrees with the

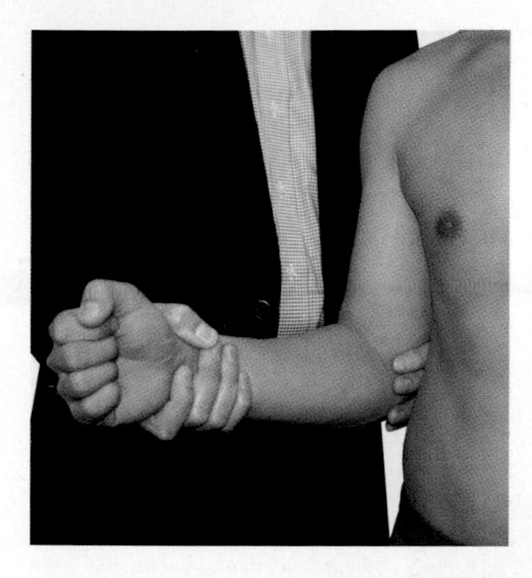

Figure 4–20 Subscapularis (C5, C6) assessment: Have the patient internally rotate his or her arm while the forearm is flexed. Stabilize the elbow at the patient's flank.

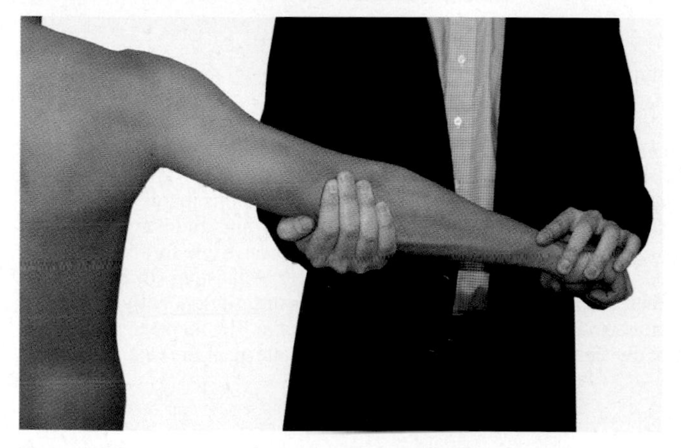

Figure 4–21 Teres major (C5, C6) assessment: To test the teres major, begin with the straightened arm abducted horizontally with the palm down. Instruct the patient to adduct the arm against resistance while you inspect the teres major.

palm facing forward (**Fig. 4–22**). In summary, all of the branches from the posterior cord act to adduct and internally rotate the arm, a point worth remembering.

♦ Brachial Plexus Divisions and the Complete Picture

Previous chapters reviewed the median, ulnar, and radial nerves. This section discussed the remaining branches of the brachial plexus, including the

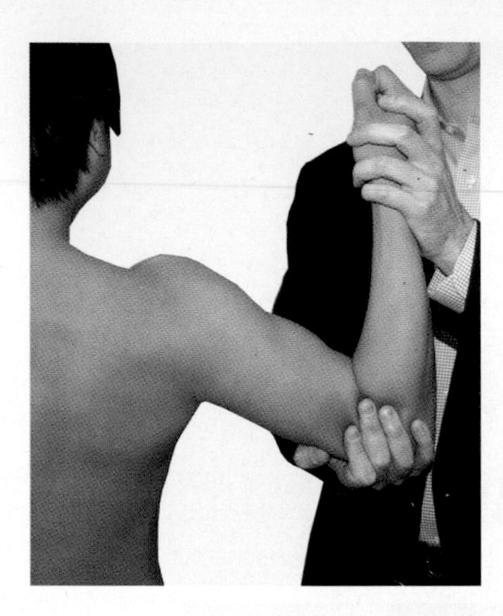

Figure 4–22 Latissimus dorsi (C6-C8) assessment: To assess the latissimus dorsi, have the patient adduct the arm when the forearm is flexed 90 degrees with the palm facing forward.

musculocutaneous and axillary nerves, as well as several more minor branches. The hard part is over; connecting the proximal and distal ends of the plexus is easy.

The brachial plexus divisions connect the trunks to the cords (**Fig. 4–23**). There are no distinct branches from the divisions. Each of the three trunks has both an anterior and posterior division. All three posterior divisions merge to create the posterior cord. The anterior divisions from the upper and middle trunks create the lateral cord; only the anterior division of the lower trunk forms the medial cord. The posterior cord receives the largest number of divisions (three); this can be remembered by the fact that the posterior cord subsequently yields the largest terminal branch of the plexus, the radial nerve. The medial cord receives the anterior division of the lower trunk, which is made up of the C8 and T1 spinal

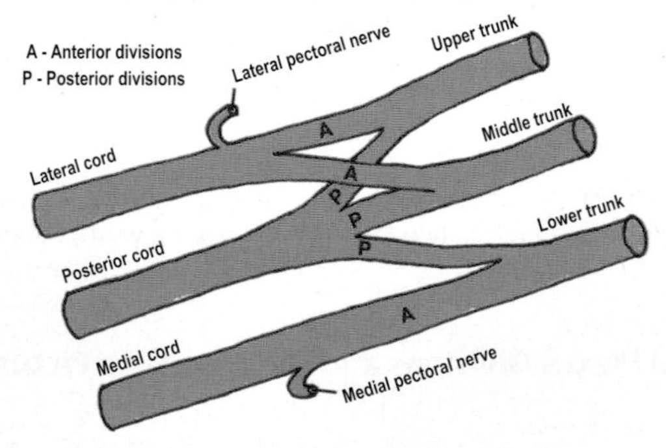

Figure 4–23 Brachial plexus divisions. The posterior cord is made up of all three posterior divisions, the lateral cord from the anterior divisions of the upper and middle trunks, and the medial cord from the lower trunk's anterior division.

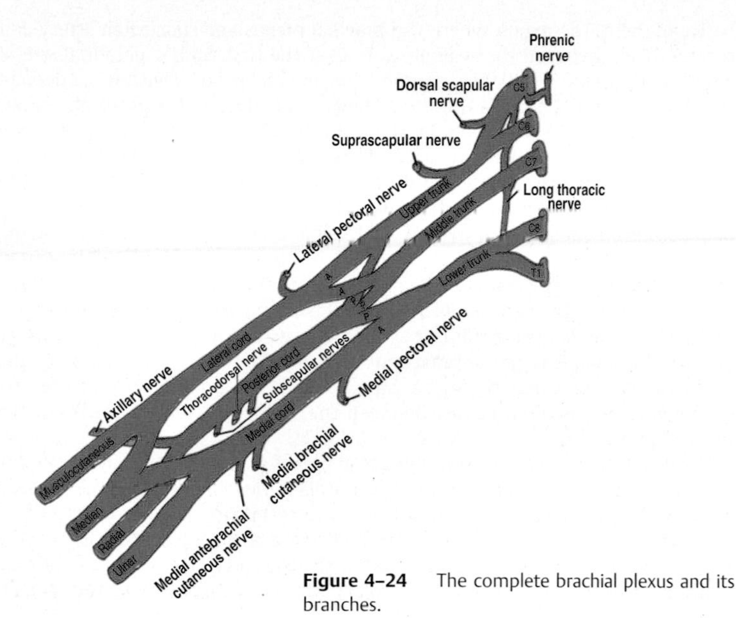

Figure 4–24 The complete brachial plexus and its branches.

nerves. Knowing that the ulnar nerve is predominantly C8 and T1, it makes sense that the medial cord, which continues distally as the ulnar nerve, originates from the anterior division of the lower trunk (**Fig. 4–24**).

- **The ulnar nerve can also have a C7 contribution. In this case, a more distal, accessory communication from the lateral cord to the ulnar nerve is usual present, which carries the C7 input.**

♦ Regional Anatomical Relationships

The brachial plexus runs in a linear path from the intervertebral foramina, under the clavicle, through the axilla, finally ending in the medial arm as terminal branches. It is intimately associated with numerous muscular, arterial, and venous structures as it passes through these regions.

The proximal brachial plexus is located within the posterior triangle of the neck. The posterior triangle of the neck is defined by the sternocleidomastoid muscle anteriorly, the trapezius posteriorly, and by the clavicle inferiorly. The posterior belly of the omohyoid traverses the lower aspect of the posterior triangle, converging with the suprascapular nerve at the scapula.

The brachial plexus runs through the interscalene triangle, which is bordered by the anterior scalene, the middle scalene, and the first rib. The apex of the interscalene triangle is located in the posterior triangle of the neck. The anterior and middle scalenes originate from the anterior and posterior tubercles, respectively, of the cervical transverse processes. These muscles run down and attach along the first rib, with the spinal nerves and brachial plexus being sandwiched between them. The region where the brachial plexus and subclavian artery exit together from between the scalenes and over the first rib is a potential site of entrapment (thoracic outlet syndrome). The brachial plexus divisions lie deep to the clavicle, while the cords and their branches are deep to the pectoralis minor and coracoid process. In the axilla, the distal brachial plexus cords lie between the clavipectoral fascia (superficial) and subscapularis muscle (deep).

The subclavian vessels exit the thorax through the ring of the first rib. The anterior scalene runs between the subclavian artery and vein, with the artery being posterior and adjacent to the C8, T1 spinal nerves and lower trunk, and the vein anterior to the anterior scalene, just deep to the clavicle. Originating from the subclavian artery soon after it emerges from the thorax, two small arterial branches traverse the surface of the brachial plexus across the posterior triangle of the neck. The more superior one is the transverse (superficial) cervical artery and the lower one is the suprascapular artery. The latter joins up with the suprascapular nerve near the suprascapular notch. A third artery, called the *dorsal scapular artery*, often passes between the upper and middle trunks of the brachial plexus.

The blood supply to the proximal brachial plexus is from the subclavian system. Specifically, the vertebral and ascending cervical arteries supply C5 and C6, the deep cervical artery irrigates C7, and the superior intercostal arteries cover C8 and T1.

As expected, the venous anatomy surrounding the brachial plexus is variable. The subclavian vein runs anterior to the anterior scalene and receives the axillary vein, which runs medial and ventral to the axillary artery in the axilla. The posterior cord

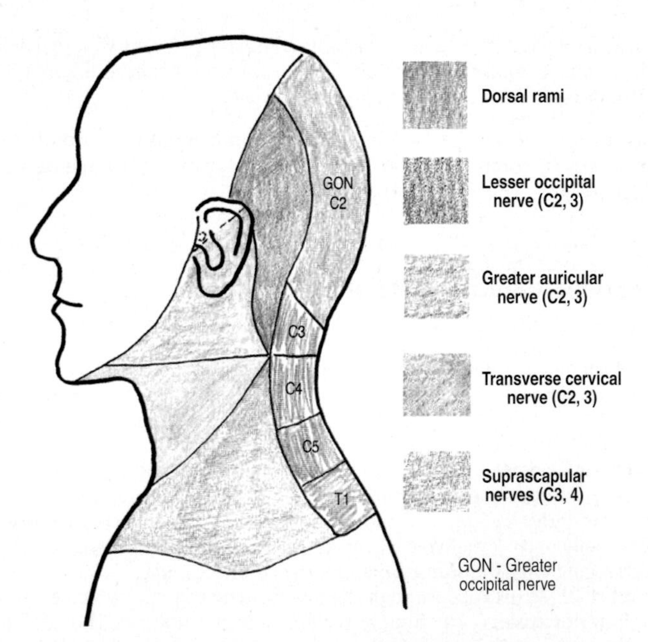

Figure 4–25 Head and neck sensory coverage, excluding the face. Sensory branches from the cervical plexus, along with the dorsal rami of the upper cervical spinal nerves, provide innervation to this area. Of note, the greater occipital nerve is made up solely of the dorsal rami of C2, and is not considered a branch of the cervical plexus.

lies deep to these two vessels. The external jugular vein drains into the subclavian vein under the clavicular attachment of the sternocleidomastoid. The external jugular vein, in general, begins at the angle of the jaw, and runs toward the shoulder by crossing the lower, anterior aspect of the posterior triangle. It runs deep to the platysma, and occasionally deep to the posterior belly of the omohyoid.

♦ The Cervical Plexus

The other plexus of the neck, the *cervical plexus*, is made up of the ventral rami of C1 to C4. After emerging from their respective intervertebral foramina, these ventral rami merge and communicate with each other, ultimately yielding several deep (motor) and superficial (sensory) branches, which originate underneath the sternocleidomastoid muscle.

The deep branches remain under the sternocleidomastoid, innervating various neck muscles (scalenes, strap muscles, levator scapula, etc.). The *ansa cervicalis* innervates the strap muscles of the neck, and is derived from these deep motor branches. The superior loop of the ansa cervicalis is made from the C1 and C2 ventral rami, while the inferior loop is from C2 and C3. The superior and inferior loops of the ansa cervicalis join anteriorly to the jugular vein.

In contrast to the deep branches, the superficial branches of the cervical plexus pour over (around and superficial to) the posterior edge of the sternocleidomastoid muscle to provide sensory coverage from the neck down to the shoulder and upper chest, including the area just below the clavicle (**Fig. 4–25**). Four named sensory branches originate from the cervical plexus, from superior to inferior: the lesser occipital, greater auricular, transverse cervical, and supraclavicular (**Fig. 4–26**). The only nerve from the cervical plexus that crosses the posterior triangle of the neck is the supraclavicular nerve and its terminal branches. If one follows the great auricular nerve back to the point where it emerges from below the sternocleidomastoid muscle, the spinal accessory nerve can often be located just a few millimeters more cranial to this point.

♦ **The greater occipital nerve originates from the *dorsal* ramus of C2. C1 provides no sensation to the skin. The *spinal accessory nerve* (CN XI) crosses the most-cranial aspect of the neck's posterior triangle.**

♦ Spinal Accessory Nerve (CN XI)

The *spinal accessory nerve* is made up of intraspinal branches from C1 to C4, and the medulla. These branches merge intradurally, with the nerve, once formed, exiting the skull base via the jugular foramen. Its relationship to the jugular vein just below the skull base is variable. After the spinal accessory nerve innervates the sternocleidomastoid muscle, which is also innervated by deep motor branches of the cervical plexus, it exits from below the sternocleidomastoid and enters the posterior triangle of the neck, approximately 8 cm superior to the clavicle. The spinal accessory nerve travels toward the top of the shoulder, eventually passing under the trapezius muscle, which it innervates (**Fig. 4–26**). As mentioned previously, this nerve commonly emerges from under the sternocleidomastoid muscle just cranial to the greater auricular nerve, the latter being an excellent surgical landmark. Across the posterior triangle, the spinal accessory nerve is interwoven with a major chain of lymph nodes. For this reason, the most common cause of isolated spinal accessory nerve palsy is iatrogenic injury following cervical lymph node dissection or biopsy. Alternatively, a painful, idiopathic spinal accessory neuropathy may also occur, which is thought to be a variant of acute brachial plexitis. *Vernet syndrome* consists of spinal accessory, vagus, and glossopharyngeal damage

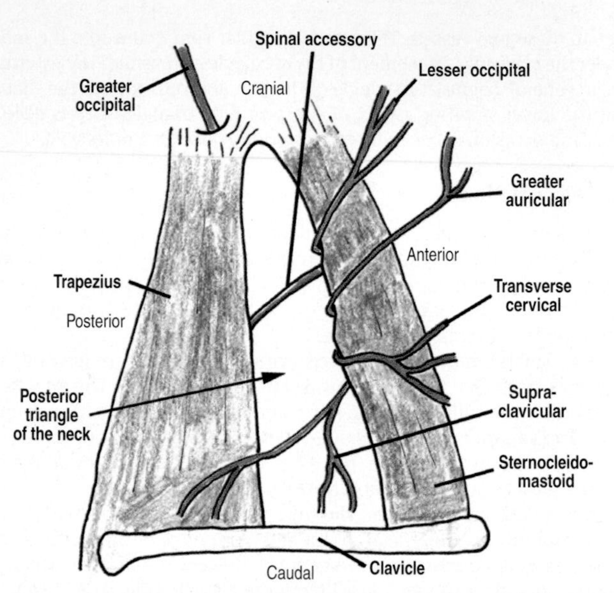

Figure 4–26 Cervical plexus and spinal accessory nerve (schematic). Four named sensory branches originate from the cervical plexus, from superior to inferior: the lesser occipital, greater auricular, transverse cervical, and supraclavicular. The only sensory nerve from the cervical plexus that crosses the posterior triangle of the neck is the supraclavicular nerve. The spinal accessory nerve emerges from under the sternocleidomastoid just a few millimeters cranially to the greater auricular nerve.

at the jugular foramen, through which all three of these nerves pass. This syndrome is usually from a local metastatic deposit or schwannoma.

A spinal accessory nerve palsy causes trapezial weakness. A patient with a weak trapezius will report trouble abducting the arm above the head (laterally), as well as shoulder girdle discomfort. Upward rotation of the scapula, mediated by the trapezius, assists the deltoid in abducting the arm above 90 degrees. Discomfort is thought to be from stress to muscles and ligaments that compensate for the trapezial weakness. At rest, the affected shoulder often lies lower than the unaffected one. Even with a complete trapezial palsy, shoulder shrug weakness seldom occurs. This is because the levator scapula muscle also shrugs the shoulder (innervated by the C3 and C4 via the cervical plexus). Weakness of the sternocleidomastoid muscle is rare, not only because the motor branches from the spinal accessory nerve branch quite proximally, but also because this muscle receives co-innervation from the cervical plexus.

Secondary to the trapezial weakness, a spinal accessory palsy also causes scapular winging. Trapezial winging is mild at rest and usually involves the upper border of the scapula, although this is variable. All types of winging (serratus anterior, trapezial, and rhomboid) are worse when the arm (partially flexed at the elbow) is pushed across the chest or in front of the body against resistance. However, only serratus anterior weakness causes winging when an extended, protracted arm is resisted. The presence of rhomboid weakness helps differentiate rhomboid versus trapezial winging. **Table 4–1** compares the three muscular causes of scapular winging.

Table 4–1 Scapular Winging: Differential Diagnosis

Nerve	Muscle	Scapular position at rest	Arm flexion	Arm abduction	Other
Long thoracic	Serratus anterior	Prominent inferomedial border	Causes winging		Winging when arm protracted
		Displaced medial	Difficulty >60 degrees		
		Rotated downward			
Spinal accessory	Trapezius	Displaced lateral		Causes winging	Shoulder hangs lower
				Difficulty >90 degrees	Trapezial atrophy
Dorsal scapular	Rhomboids	Prominent inferomedial border			Rhomboid weakness
		Displaced lateral			Rhomboid atrophy
		Rotated upward			

5

Clinical Evaluation of the Brachial Plexus

Before attempting to examine patients with injuries to the brachial plexus, one should fully understand brachial plexus anatomy. The proper examination techniques for the muscles of the upper extremity and shoulder girdle must also be mastered. In this chapter, I will present this often-daunting anatomical information, discuss lesion localization in the brachial plexus, and provide guidelines for examining patients. The clinical aspects of some common causes of brachial plexus injury will also be described; these should be kept in mind when formulating a differential diagnosis.

♦ The Proximal Brachial Plexus Palsies

Spinal Nerve Myotomes

Like spinal nerve dermatomes, spinal nerve myotomes are *approximations*. Despite variations, however, learning spinal nerve myotomes remains important for the clinical evaluation of patients with cervical radiculopathies and proximal brachial plexus lesions. The C5 to T1 spinal nerve myotomes are presented below.

The C5 Spinal Nerve: Arm Raise

The semi-autonomous muscular innervation of the C5 spinal nerve includes arm abduction and external rotation. These two movements are very important for upper extremity function and are classically lost following an upper brachial plexus injury (e.g., birth palsy). The terminal branches mediating these movements include the axillary nerve to the deltoid muscle, and the suprascapular nerve to the supraspinatus and infraspinatus muscles. The supraspinatus (first 30 degrees) and deltoid (30 to 90 degrees) abduct the arm; the infraspinatus is the arm's most important external rotator (the teres major also externally rotates the arm). A composite movement involving all three of these muscles, and therefore predominantly mediated by the C5 nerve root, is the arm raise. Beginning with the arms straight along the side of the body, the patient abducts them to 90 degrees, while simultaneously externally rotating them so that the undersurface of the upper arm faces forward (**Fig. 5–1**).

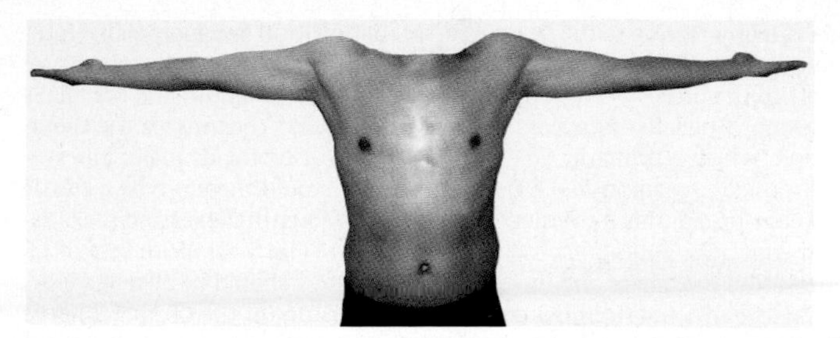

Figure 5–1 Semi-autonomous motor innervation of the C5 spinal nerve: the arm raise. Beginning with the arms straight along the sides of the body, the patient simultaneously abducts and externally rotates the arms to 90 degrees.

The C5 dermatome covers the lateral portion of the shoulder and arm down to the elbow (**Fig. 5–2**). In part, the upper-lateral cutaneous nerve to the axillary nerve, as well as the lower-lateral brachial cutaneous nerve to the proximal radial nerve carries sensation from this area.

The C6 Spinal Nerve: Chin-up

The semi-autonomous muscular innervation of the C6 spinal nerve includes forearm supination and flexion, as well as arm extension and adduction. The radial

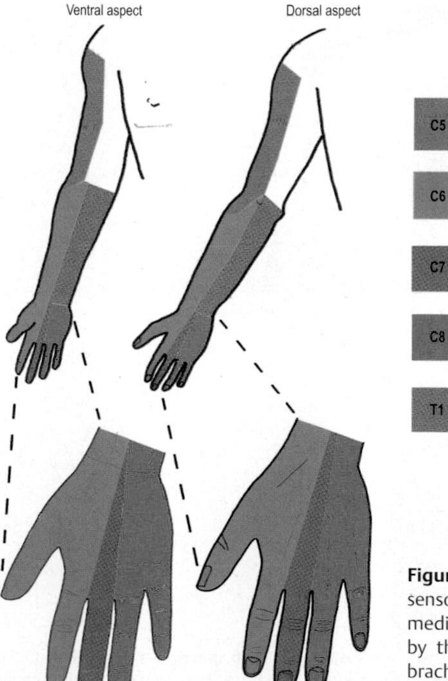

Figure 5–2 Upper extremity (C5-T1) sensory dermatomes. Sensation to the medial upper arm (not shaded) is carried by the T2 spinal nerve via the medial brachial cutaneous nerve.

nerve caries C6 innervation to the supinator (supination) and brachioradialis (forearm flexion with the forearm partially supinated). The musculocutaneous nerve carries fibers to the biceps brachii (forearm flexion and supination) and brachialis (forearm flexion). The latissimus dorsi extends and adducts the arm via the thoracodorsal nerve, which is primarily C6 mediated (C7 can also provide major innervation to this muscle). A composite C6 body movement would therefore be a classic underhand chin-up. For this movement, the supinated forearm flexes and the latissimus dorsi contracts, pulling one's chin over the bar (**Fig. 5–3**). With loss of C6 motor innervation the biceps and brachioradialis reflexes should be absent.

The lateral forearm and thumb are the sensory territory of the C6 spinal nerve (**Fig. 5–2**). This sensation is carried in part by the lateral antebrachial cutaneous nerve to the musculocutaneous nerve, and for the thumb, by the terminal sensory branches of both the median and radial nerves.

The Upper Trunk

The upper trunk carries axons from the C5 and C6 spinal nerves. Injury to the upper trunk is commonly caused when the shoulder is forced downward, while the head is simultaneously stabilized or pushed in the opposite direction,

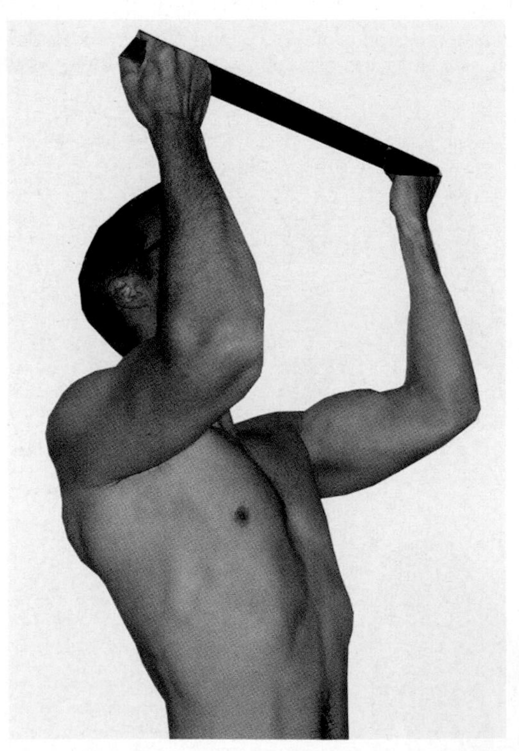

Figure 5–3 Semi-autonomous motor innervation of the C6 spinal nerve: the chin-up. For this movement, the supinated forearm flexes, and the latissimus dorsi contracts; this pulls the chin over the bar.

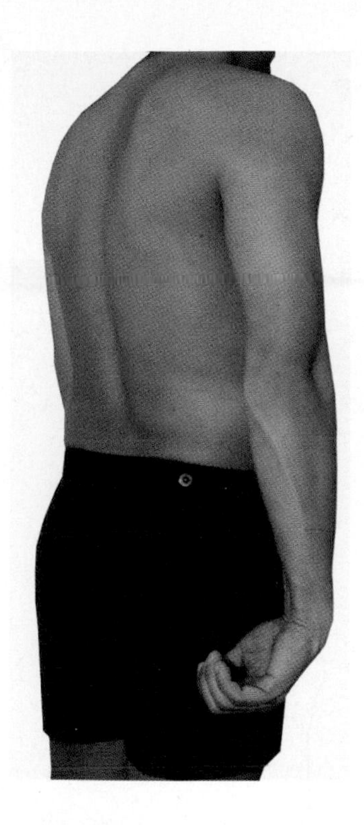

Figure 5–4 Erb's palsy or waiter's tip position waiter's (simulated). Patients characteristically have the affected arm adducted and internally rotated (unopposed pull of pectoralis major), forearm extended and pronated (unopposed pull of the triceps and pronator teres), and the wrist and fingers flexed (from weak finger and wrist extensors [variable C6 innervation]).

thereby stretching the upper portion of the brachial plexus. This mechanism of injury commonly occurs with motorcycle trauma, falls, and birth palsies. An upper trunk injury is referred to as an *Erb's palsy*. With this injury, the C5 and C6 innervated muscles are weak. The affected limb assumes a characteristic position at rest secondary to the unopposed action of the remaining musculature. Patients typically have their affected arm adducted and internally rotated (unopposed pull of pectoralis major), forearm extended and pronated (unopposed pull of the triceps and pronator teres), and the wrist and fingers flexed (from weak finger and wrist extensors [variable C6 innervation]). This position is called the *waiter's tip position* (**Fig. 5–4**).

The same mechanisms may cause either an upper trunk or spinal nerve injury. However, weakness involving the rhomboids (dorsal scapular nerve), serratus anterior (long thoracic nerve), and/or diaphragm (phrenic nerve), helps localize the injury to the C5 and C6 spinal nerves, where these branches originate, rather than the upper trunk per se. A lesion involving the upper trunk, or alternatively both the C5 and C6 spinal nerves, causes sensory loss on the lateral half of the arm and forearm, as well as the whole thumb (**Fig. 5–5**).

The Middle Trunk

The C7 Spinal Nerve: Triceps Push Down

The middle trunk is only made up of fibers from the C7 spinal nerve; hence, these two neural elements will be considered together. The near autonomous muscular

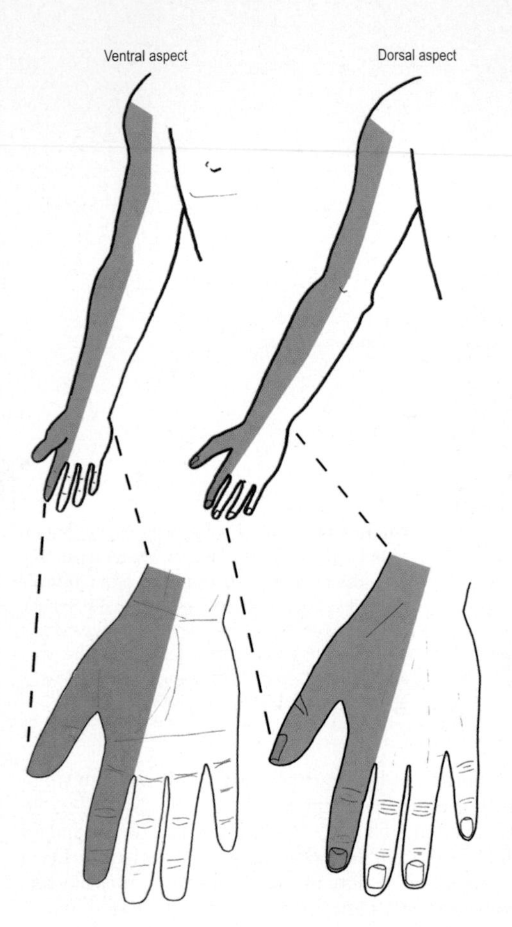

Figure 5–5 Sensory loss for an upper trunk or combination C5/C6 spinal nerve injury. This lesion yields a sensory loss involving the lateral half of the arm and forearm, as well as the whole thumb.

control of the C7 nerve root includes the triceps (radial nerve), flexor carpi radialis (median nerve), flexor carpi ulnaris (ulnar nerve), and pronator teres (median nerve). C7 also provides innervation to the wrist extensors, finger extensors, and finger flexors. However, innervation of the latter muscles is either variable, or strongly shared with other nerve roots (e.g., C6, C8); therefore, they are not considered autonomous. The composite movement of the C7 spinal nerve and middle trunk is the triceps pushdown. This movement is made, for example, when you push down on a tabletop when getting up from being seated at a table (**Fig. 5–6**). For this to occur, one places the forearms in pronation (pronator teres), flexes the wrists (flexor carpi radialis and ulnaris), and contracts the triceps to extend the forearms. A person with a middle trunk palsy cannot do this. It is not possible to differentiate a middle trunk from C7 spinal nerve lesion based on motor examination alone. To do so, one must use other clinical and radiographic findings (e.g., C7 sensory nerve action potential, myelography, spinal nerve lesions present at adjacent levels, etc.).

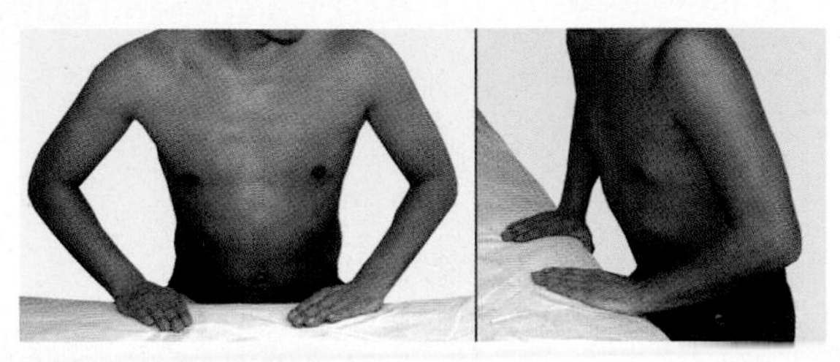

Figure 5–6 Semi-autonomous motor innervation of the C7 spinal nerve: Triceps press down. This movement is made when you push down on a tabletop upon getting up from being seated. For this to occur, one places the forearm in pronation (pronator teres), flexes the wrist (flexor carpi radialis), and contracts the triceps to extend the forearms.

The volar and dorsal aspects of the long finger are almost exclusively within the C7 dermatome (**Fig. 5–2**). The sensory division of the median nerve (volar aspect of the long finger and its nail bed) and the superficial sensory radial nerve (dorsal aspect of the long finger) carry this sensation. Lesions of the middle trunk, made up solely of C7 fibers, logically cause the same pattern of sensory loss as does a pure C7 palsy.

The C8 Spinal Nerve: Hand Grasp

The C8 spinal nerve provides motor input to many of the long finger flexors (and extensors), as well as to the hand intrinsic muscles, sharing the innervation of this latter group of muscles with T1. Some of the most common muscles to become weak with a C8 palsy include the flexor profundi to the index and long finger (distal interphalangeal joint flexion), thenar intrinsics including the abductor pollicis brevis and opponens pollicis, and extensors to the thumb, forefinger, and long finger. Therefore, an easy way to assess C8 function is to have the patient grasp *and let go* of your fingers, with special attention paid to the first three digits (**Fig. 5–7**). A C8 palsy would prevent the patient from performing this movement accurately and strongly.

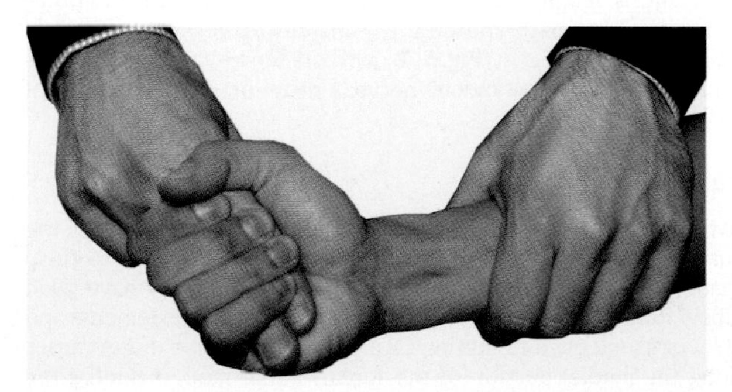

Figure 5–7 Semi-autonomous motor innervation of the C8 spinal nerve: hand grasp. A quick and easy way to assess C8 function is to have the patient grasp *and let go* of your fingers, with attention paid especially to the first three digits. A patient with a C8 palsy will have trouble doing this smoothly, strongly, and repetitively.

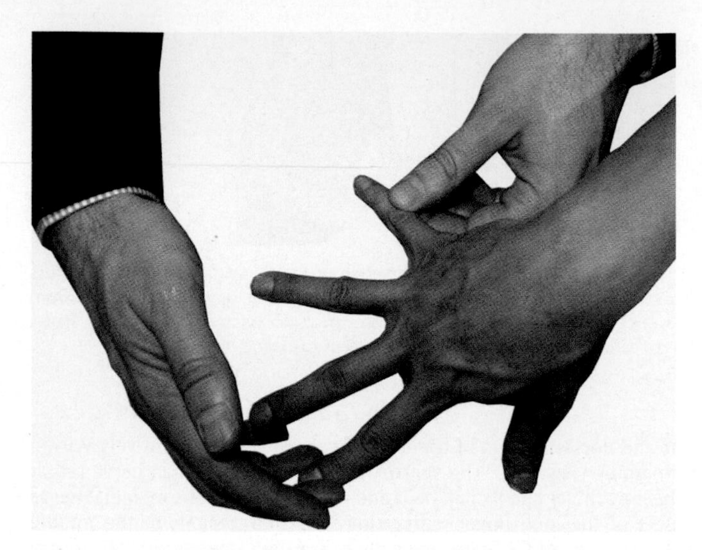

Figure 5–8 Semi-autonomous motor innervation of the T1 spinal nerve: spreading the fingers. The T1 spinal nerve is best tested in isolation by having the patient spread the fingers. The dorsal interossei muscles control this movement. Atrophy of the first dorsal interosseus muscle, when present, is readily observed.

The C8 dermatome covers the medial, or ulnar, third of the hand, including the fifth digit and lateral hypothenar eminence (**Fig. 5–2**). The dorsal ulnar cutaneous and palmar ulnar cutaneous nerves, along with the superficial sensory division of the ulnar nerve, carry sensation from this area.

The T1 Spinal Nerve: Spreading the Fingers

The T1 spinal nerve is best tested in near isolation by having the patient spread the fingers (**Fig. 5–8**). This movement is mediated by the dorsal interossei muscles, which are predominantly T1 innervated. Atrophy of the first dorsal interosseus muscle, when present, is readily observed. The ulnar nerve carries T1 motor fibers down to the dorsal interossei muscles. The T1 sensory dermatome mainly covers the medial half of the forearm (**Fig. 5–2**), with its sensory fibers being carried by the medial antebrachial cutaneous nerve, a distal branch of the medial cord.

The Lower Trunk

Because the lower trunk is made up of the C8 and T1 nerve roots, injuries of the lower trunk cause marked hand weakness, including problems with hand grasp and finger spreading. Patients with lower trunk injuries classically have good shoulder and elbow function, but report trouble with fine finger movements and grip strength. A lower trunk or combination C8 and T1 spinal nerve lesion causes sensory loss along the medial portion of the forearm and hand, including the fifth digit (**Fig. 5–9**).

Injury to both the C8 and T1 spinal nerves is called a *Klumpke's palsy*. This injury may occur with violent upward pulling of a child's outstretched arm, or following any type of injury where the upper extremity is suddenly forced upward (e.g.,

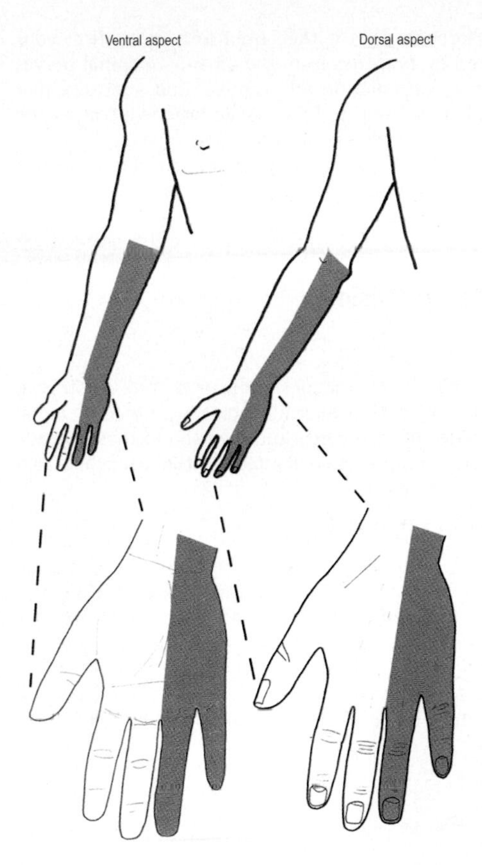

Figure 5–9 Sensory loss for a lower trunk or C8/T1 spinal nerve lesion. This lesion causes a sensory loss in the medial portion of the forearm and hand, including the fifth digit.

grabbing something when falling, motorcycle accidents). Birth palsy may rarely present as an isolated Klumpke's paralysis.

Pancoast syndrome is invasion and compression of the lower trunk by an apical lung mass. It usually begins with pain radiating down the inner aspect of the arm and forearm. Approximately one third of patients develop motor and sensory deficits, and two thirds have Horner's syndrome. Small tumors can be undetectable on X-ray; therefore, a computerized tomography (CT) scan with contrast is often required to confirm the diagnosis.

- **The medial arm is predominantly covered by the T2 dermatome. The T3 dermatome includes the axilla and a portion of the proximal, medial arm.**

Summary

Assessment of the proximal brachial plexus (spinal nerves and trunks) should be performed with an understanding of spinal nerve myotomes. Patterns of muscular weakness are used to localize the injury to one or more of the spinal nerves or trunks. Sensory loss of the upper lateral arm (C5), thumb (C6), long finger (C7), fifth finger (C8), and medial forearm (T1) is then used to help confirm your localization. Muscles innervated by branches from the C5 and C6 spinal nerves and upper trunk (long thoracic, phrenic, dorsal scapular, and suprascapular nerves) may be examined and then used to differentiate lesions affecting the upper trunk versus spinal nerves. Supplemental information useful for lesion localization includes myelography to document pseudomeningoceles, and chest radiographs to evaluate diaphragm asymmetry.

♦ The Distal Brachial Plexus Palsies

Plus Palsies

The easiest way to remember the clinical manifestations of a cord lesion is to think of what happens to a patient with a musculocutaneous, ulnar, or radial nerve palsy (the terminal branches of each cord), and then add to these nerve's respective patterns of weakness any muscles innervated by other branches from the cord in question. I call these *plus palsies*.

Lateral Cord: Musculocutaneous Plus *Palsy*

The lateral cord is formed by the anterior divisions of both upper and middle trunks, and therefore, contains fibers from C5, C6, and C7. This cord bifurcates providing the median nerve's lateral component (C5 to C7), and then continues distally as the musculocutaneous nerve. As expected, an isolated lesion to the lateral cord consists of a musculocutaneous nerve palsy, *plus* a partial median nerve deficit; that is, a deficit only involving the median nerve's C5 to C7 portion. This deficit pattern may be termed a *musculocutaneous* plus *palsy* (**Fig. 5–10**).

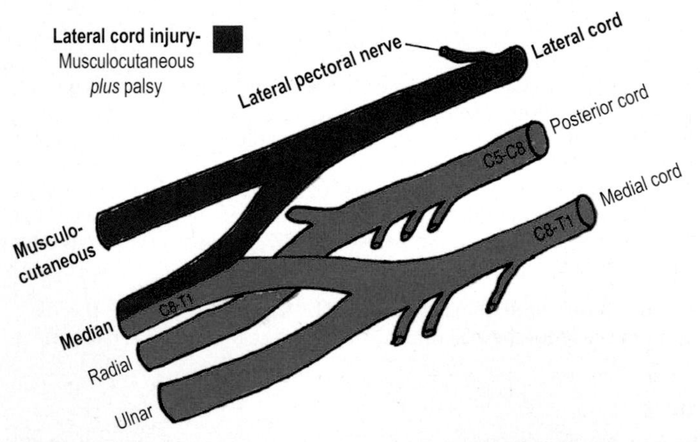

Figure 5–10 Musculocutaneous *plus* palsy (lateral cord injury). The lateral cord terminates by providing the median nerve's lateral component (C5-C7), and then continues distally as the musculocutaneous nerve. As expected, an isolated lesion to the lateral cord consists of a musculocutaneous nerve palsy *plus* a partial median nerve deficit involving its C5 to C7 portion.

The classic musculocutaneous palsy causes forearm flexion weakness secondary to biceps brachii, coracobrachialis, and brachialis weakness, and sensory loss in the lateral forearm (lateral antebrachial cutaneous nerve). As mentioned, median nerve function can be divided into lateral (C5 to C7; lateral cord) and medial (C8, T1; medial cord) components. The lateral cord provides all the median nerve's sensory fibers (the medial cord does not provide cutaneous sensation to the median nerve). Therefore, lateral palm and first three digit sensory loss occurs with a lateral cord injury. Although the lateral component is primarily sensory, it also controls the more proximal median innervated muscles (pronator teres and flexor carpi radialis). In contrast, the medial (C8, T1) component controls the distal median innervated muscles (hand intrinsics). The long finger flexors (flexor digitorum superficialis and the flexor digitorum profundus to the first two fingers) represent an intermediate gray zone, with contribution from both median nerve components. However, the C8 and T1 contribution is usually greater for these muscles.

Therefore, a lateral cord injury causes a musculocutaneous palsy (forearm flexion weakness), *plus* forearm pronation and wrist flexion weakness secondary to involvement of the lateral cord's motor contribution to the median nerve. Sensory loss in the lateral forearm and tips of the first three digits should also be present following a lateral cord injury. Furthermore, weakness of the clavicular head of the pectoralis major should also occur, considering the medial pectoral nerve, which innervates this muscle, originates from the lateral cord.

Medial Cord: Ulnar **Plus** *Palsy*

The medial cord is a continuation of the lower trunk's anterior division, containing C8 and T1 nerve fibers. Although an accessory branch from the lateral cord donating some C7 fibers can occur, this is omitted for simplicity. The medial cord provides the medial component of the median nerve, containing C8 and T1 fibers, and then continues as the ulnar nerve into the arm. Therefore, an isolated medial cord lesion consists of an ulnar nerve palsy, *plus* the loss of C8/T1 median nerve function (**Fig. 5–11**).

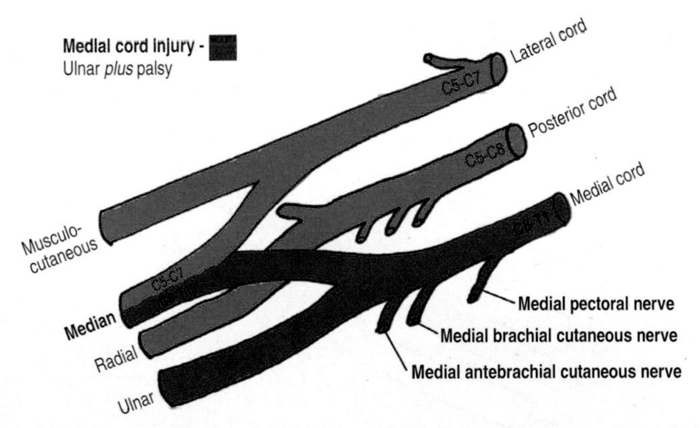

Figure 5–11 Ulnar *plus* palsy (medial cord injury). The medial cord provides the medial root to the median nerve, containing C8 and T1 fibers, and then continues as the ulnar nerve into the arm. Therefore, an isolated medial cord lesion consists of an ulnar nerve palsy *plus* weakness in the muscles controlled by the C8 and T1 components of the median nerve.

An ulnar palsy causes weakness in medial wrist flexion (flexor carpi ulnaris), distal interphalangeal joint flexion weakness involving the fourth and fifth digits (flexor digitorum profundus), other fifth digit movements (opponens, flexor, and abductor digiti minimi), and finger abduction and adduction (interossei). Ulnar nerve sensory loss involves the medial third of the hand. As mentioned, the medial component of the median nerve controls the median nerve innervated hand intrinsics, including the opponens pollicis, flexor pollicis brevis (superficial head), abductor pollicis brevis, and the first two lumbricals. Therefore, a medial cord lesion, or ulnar *plus* palsy, would in addition to causing ulnar motor loss, cause median innervated thumb weakness, as well as difficulty extending the proximal interphalangeal joints of the first two fingers (lumbricals). Of note, these C8/T1 median nerve muscles are the same ones whose innervation is exchanged with a Martin–Gruber anastomosis (see Chapter 1).

The medial cord also has a few side branches that can be tested to confirm medial cord involvement. The medial brachial and antebrachial cutaneous nerves originate from the distal medial cord and mediate sensation over the medial aspect of the arm and forearm, respectively. The medial pectoral nerve originates from the proximal medial cord, and if damaged, causes weakness in the sternal head of the pectoralis major.

Posterior Cord: Radial Plus *Palsy*

The posterior cord is made up of the posterior division of all three trunks, containing input from C5 to C8. The presence of T1 fibers in the posterior cord is controversial and, needless to say, variable. The terminal branches of the posterior cord are the radial and axillary nerves; therefore, a combination palsy of these two nerves is the hallmark of a posterior cord injury (**Fig. 5–12**). Hence, a posterior cord injury may also be called a *radial-axillary palsy* or *radial* plus *palsy*.

A radial palsy causes weakness in forearm extension (triceps), forearm supination (supinator), wrist extension (extensor carpi radialis longus and brevis, extensor carpi ulnaris), and finger/thumb extension (superficial and deep finger extensors). Radial nerve sensory loss involves the posterior arm (posterior brachial cutaneous nerve) and forearm (posterior antebrachial cutaneous nerve), the lower lateral

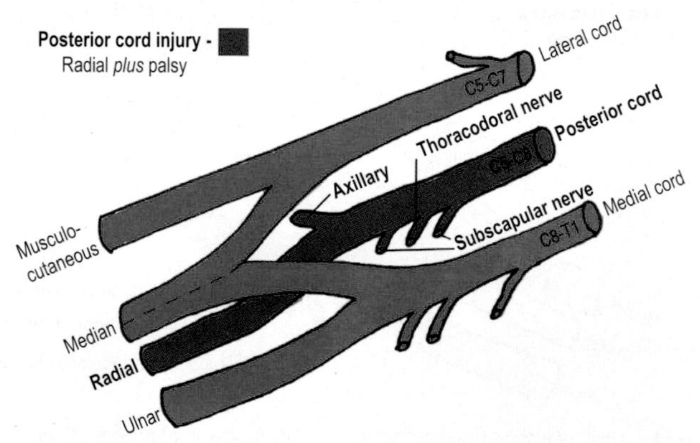

Figure 5–12 Radial *plus* palsy (radial-axillary palsy, posterior cord injury). The two terminal branches of the posterior cord are the radial and axillary nerves; therefore, a combination palsy of these two nerves is the hallmark of a posterior cord injury.

aspect of the arm (lower lateral brachial cutaneous nerve), and the dorsolateral hand (superficial sensory radial nerve). An axillary palsy causes arm abduction weakness secondary to deltoid paralysis. An axillary nerve lesion can also cause sensory loss in the upper lateral arm (upper lateral brachial cutaneous nerve), especially if the patient is examined soon after injury. Furthermore, arm adduction and internal rotation weakness helps confirm posterior cord damage because the minor branches off the posterior cord control these movements (i.e., the upper and lower subscapular, and thoracodorsal nerves).

Summary

To assess the distal brachial plexus, one needs to be familiar with patterns of neurological deficits that may occur following injury to its terminal branches: the musculocutaneous, median, ulnar, radial, and axillary nerves. With this knowledge, diagnosis of cord-level injuries becomes straightforward; cord injuries cause deficits that are a combination of those seen with injury to their branches. Therefore, analogous to proximal brachial plexus injury being assessed by referring to its spinal nerve components, the distal plexus is evaluated by using knowledge of its major terminal branches.

♦ Assessment of Divisional Injuries

Isolated injury to one of the brachial plexus divisions can be difficult to differentiate clinically from cord- or trunk-level lesions. Furthermore, it is usually not possible to say if divisions are damaged in addition to cords or trunks without surgical exploration.

An isolated injury to one, or more, divisions yields neurological deficits that are the same, or less severe, than a cord-level injury. For example, an injury to the anterior division of the lower trunk (C8/T1) should involve nearly all the fibers in the medial cord. However, a divisional injury affecting the lateral cord may only involve the anterior division from the upper trunk (C5/C6) or the anterior division from the middle trunk (C7). Injury to any of the three posterior divisions will cause a partial posterior cord deficit. For example, an isolated injury to the posterior division of the upper trunk may be confused with an axillary nerve palsy; however, presence of some brachioradialis and supinator weakness, along with sensory loss on the dorsal thumb (C6 dermatome via superficial sensory radial nerve) should point to a partial cord or divisional injury rather than an axillary nerve palsy.

With an ability to readily diagnose proximal and distal brachial plexus lesions, one can deduce a divisional injury. Nevertheless divisional lesions may be indistinguishable from partial cord injuries. Fortunately, injuries only involving the divisions are infrequent.

♦ Diagnosis of Preganglionic Injury

Many stretch injuries to the brachial plexus actually cause avulsion of the ventral and dorsal rootlets from the spinal cord itself. The C8 and T1 spinal rootlets are most prone to this type of injury because these spinal nerves have minimal anchoring to their respective troughs along the transverse processes. In contrast, the C5 to C6 spinal nerves are strongly attached to their respective transverse processes, thereby making avulsion at these levels less likely when a similar force is applied. There are multiple ways to determine if a spinal root has a preganglionic, or avulsion, injury, which is very important for prognosis and treatment.

Myelography supplemented with postmyelography CT scanning has good sensitivity in detecting pseudomeningoceles and absent (avulsed) nerve rootlets at each cervical level. These two findings are highly suggestive of rootlet avulsion. Magnetic resonance imaging (MRI) may also be used to document these findings; however, most medical centers do not routinely provide images of adequate resolution. Involvement of very proximal branches of the brachial plexus, including the phrenic nerve (paralyzed diaphragm), dorsal scapular nerve (rhomboid weakness), and long thoracic nerve (scapular winging) also suggests preganglionic damage, or at least intraforaminal damage. Avulsion of the T1 spinal nerve can cause Horner's syndrome, the presence of which should be documented.

Electrophysiological testing is also quite useful in confirming preganglionic damage. With this type of injury, the peripheral nerve sensory axons remain connected to their cell bodies in the spinal ganglia. Therefore, the amplitudes of distal extremity sensory nerve action potentials (SNAPs) remain normal (or increased), despite no sensation being present on examination. Presence of compound motor action potentials (CMAPs) argue against spinal cord avulsion.

♦ The Examination Approach

The Comprehensive Examination

When examining the brachial plexus and upper extremity, one should employ a comprehensive and systematic approach, beginning proximally and proceeding distally. With the exception of a screening assessment in the emergency department, an abbreviated or focused examination is not recommended. This is because some subtle, yet important, deficits can be missed. My examination routine is divided into six distinct steps (**Table 5–1**).

- *Step 1: The back.* The exam begins with the patient facing away from the examiner. The presence of scapular winging, muscle atrophy, and asymmetry of the shoulders and scapulae at rest are noted. Next, the patient shrugs his or her shoulders upward to assess trapezial and levator scapulae function. Having the patient bring the scapulae together assesses the rhomboids. The latissimus dorsi are palpated bilaterally and the patient is asked to cough. The patient is instructed to raise the arms to the sides and above the head to check trapezial function. Next, the patient is told to reach toward the wall with the affected arm and scapular winging is evaluated, first with the arm protracted, and then with it flexed.

- *Step 2: The shoulder.* Starting with the arm straight and to the side, the patient is instructed to abduct the arm. In doing so, the supraspinatus and deltoid are assessed. With the arm horizontal to the floor, the posterior head of the deltoid (posterior movement) and teres major (downward movement) are tested. The patient then flexes the forearm 90 degrees ("hold-up" position) and both the clavicular (lateral pectoral nerve) and sternal (medial pectoral nerve) heads of the pectoralis major are assessed, both visually and by palpation. Facing the patient's flank, external arm rotation is tested (infraspinatus).

Table 5–1 The Six Steps of a Comprehensive Brachial Plexus Examination

1 – Back
Observation
Rhomboids
Latissimus dorsi
Trapezius
Scapular winging
2 – Shoulder
Supraspinatus
Deltoid
Posterior deltoid
Teres major
Pectoralis major
Infraspinatus
3 – Arm
Triceps
Biceps
Brachioradialis
4 – Forearm
Supinator
Pronator
Wrist flexion
Wrist extension
Finger extension
5 – Hand
Observation
Finger flexion
Thenar intrinsics
Hypothenar intrinsics
Interossei
Lumbricals
6 – Skin
Sensation
Perspiration/Horner's
Pulses/masses
Reflexes/Tinel's sign

- *Step 3: The arm.* The triceps are examined with the upper arm parallel to the floor, so the effect of gravity is eliminated. Forearm flexion at the elbow is tested with the forearm fully supinated (biceps brachii) and half supinated (brachioradialis).
- *Step 4: The forearm.* Supination and pronation are tested with the elbow straight. Next, wrist movement is assessed. The patient flexes the wrist (flexor carpi radialis and ulnaris), and then the arm is pronated and the forearm extensors are tested (extensor carpi radialis longus and brevis, and extensor carpi ulnaris). With the arm placed on a flat surface, the long forearm finger extensors (extensor digitorum communis, extensor indicis, extensor digiti minimi, and extensors pollicis longus and brevis) are also evaluated.
- *Step 5: The hand.* The hand is first observed at rest for signs of atrophy. The patient should be instructed to open and close the hand so that any evidence

of contracture can be observed, if present (e.g., claw hand). Next, the thumb is evaluated further, including abduction, adduction, opposition, and flexion. The okay and Froment's signs are checked for. Flexion at the proximal (flexor digitorum superficialis) and distal (flexor digitorum profundus) interphalangeal joints is assessed. Abduction and opposition of the fifth digit is evaluated, as well as Wartenburg's and palmaris brevis signs. Finger abduction (dorsal interossei), adduction (palmar interossei), and extension at the interphalangeal joints is tested (lumbricals).

- *Step 6: The skin.* Sensation with light touch and pinprick is tested from the shoulder down to the hand. Testing is performed circumferentially on the arm, forearm, and hand. The fingertips are also tested, which is especially important considering the thumb, long finger, and fifth digit each represent a different dermatome. Any abnormality or asymmetry between the upper extremities is evaluated further, including assessment of two-point discrimination and localization. Lack of sweating may be observed with an ophthalmoscope. The neck and axilla are palpated and observed for scars, masses, or a Tinel's sign. To finish, pulses and reflexes (C6, C7) are tested.

Localization of the lesion is then performed using one's knowledge of peripheral nerve anatomy. The deficit may then be graded for both research purposes, as well as for serial assessment of improvement, or lack thereof.

The Screening Examination

In certain situations (e.g., in the emergency department or trauma slot) an abbreviated screening examination for brachial plexus injury may be indicated. This emergent evaluation, however, is often limited by other injuries, including long bone fractures, spine trauma, and patient confusion or stupor. The screening examination, or primary survey, evaluates 9 muscles that have been selected because they each follow a separate path through the brachial plexus (**Table 5–2**). These muscles include two shoulder, three arm, and four hand muscles.

This primary survey is performed with the patient supine or sitting. The following two shoulder muscles are tested: deltoid, and infraspinatus. Next, the

Table 5–2 The Brachial Plexus Screening Examination*

Shoulder		
	Deltoid	C5, upper trunk, posterior cord, axillary nerve
	Infraspinatus	C5, upper trunk, suprascapular nerve
Arm		
	Biceps	C6, upper trunk, lateral cord, musculocutaneous nerve
	Brachioradialis	C6, upper trunk, posterior cord, radial nerve
	Triceps	C7, middle trunk, posterior cord, radial nerve
Hand		
	Flexor carpi radialis	C7, middle trunk, lateral cord, median nerve
	Extensor indicis	C8, lower trunk, posterior cord, radial nerve
	Abductor pollicis brevis	C8, lower trunk, medial cord, median nerve
	Dorsal interossei	T1, lower trunk, medial cord, ulnar nerve

*The 9 muscles are assessed proximally to distally. Spinal nerve contributions are simplified.

following arm muscles are tested: biceps, brachioradialis, and triceps. Finally, hand movements are tested, including the flexor carpi radialis, extensor indicis, abductor pollicis brevis, and dorsal interossei.

If the primary survey reveals a deficit, a secondary survey in the emergency department is performed; this includes sensory and additional motor testing. The primary survey reveals if the lesion is proximal or distal. Proximal lesions are secondarily tested using a spinal nerve template (Which spinal nerves are affected?), whereas distal brachial plexus injuries are assessed with a cord approach (Which cords are affected, and to what extent?). To perform the secondary survey, think of all the muscles innervated by the injured element (as determined by the primary survey, e.g., upper trunk, medial cord) and then test them all from proximal to distal. A comprehensive examination (described previously) should always be performed; however, in most severe trauma patients, this is performed later when the patient is fully cooperative and more time is available.

♦ Processes Affecting the Brachial Plexus

Brachial plexus injuries are most often traumatic, with stretch (including birth palsies), lacerations, gunshots, and blunt contusions being the more common mechanisms. Other, less frequent etiologies include compression by anomalous fibrous ridges on the scalene musculature (neurogenic thoracic outlet syndrome), delayed radiation damage, and acute brachial plexitis (Parsonage–Turner syndrome). Considering the patient's history and risk factors, an accurate etiological diagnosis can usually be made, even before examination. Some specific causes of brachial plexus injury will be discussed.

Neurogenic Thoracic Outlet Syndrome

Symptoms of neurogenic thoracic outlet syndrome, or *Gilliat-Sumner hand*, are predominantly caused by irritation to the C8 and T1 spinal nerves, and/or lower trunk. "Disputed," arterial, and venous forms of thoracic outlet syndrome are separate clinical entities and will not be commented upon. The source of irritation for neurogenic thoracic outlet syndrome is localized to the scalene triangle. The scalene triangle is made up of the anterior scalene anteriorly, the middle scalene posteriorly, and the edge of the first rib inferiorly. The brachial plexus and subclavian artery pass through this triangle, but the subclavian vein does not. Irritation of the brachial plexus is often from an abnormal fibrous band, on or near these two scalene muscles. An elongated C7 transverse process or cervical rib may be present, both of which unfavorably re-orient the borders of the scalene muscles, possibly leading to neural compression or irritation. The patient with classic neurogenic thoracic outlet syndrome has forward drooping shoulders.

Manifestations of neurogenic thoracic outlet syndrome are usually localized to the C8 and T1 nerve roots. These patients present with progressive hand intrinsic weakness and atrophy. Sensory loss, when present, occurs on the medial aspect of the forearm, as well as on the medial third of the hand. In terms of the terminal brachial plexus branches, the hand intrinsic weakness and atrophy are often more median than ulnar, whereas the sensory loss is all ulnar (ulnar and medial antebrachial cutaneous nerves, both from the medial cord). Pain is not usually of significant concern to the patient, but a dull ache in the shoulder girdle or axilla is not uncommon. Externally rotating the arm, while abducting it above the head, often precipitates or worsens symptoms after a minute or two in this position (Roos maneuver or elevated arm stress test [EAST]). Loss of a radial pulse with this maneuver (Adson's sign) may also occur. Both of these provocative tests, however, have a high rate of false-positives; therefore, they are of limited value. A supraclavicular Tinel's sign may be present. A cervical radiograph should be ordered to rule out a cervical rib or elongated C7 transverse process.

Care must be taken to differentiate thoracic outlet syndrome from a C8 radiculopathy or ulnar compression at the elbow. Concurrent weakness in median (abductor pollicis brevis) as well as ulnar (abductor digiti minimi or the first dorsal interosseous) innervated muscles helps confirm a more proximal injury at the brachial plexus (i.e., neurogenic thoracic outlet, and not carpal or cubital tunnel syndromes). No history of neck or radicular pain, along with the presence of both C8 and T1 sensory and motor changes, helps exclude a single-level radiculopathy.

Birth-Related Brachial Plexus Palsy

Newborns can have stretch injuries to their proximal brachial plexus during difficult deliveries, vaginal or otherwise. Heavy birth weight is considered a predisposing factor. The most common injury is an *Erb's palsy*, where C5 and C6 (or the upper trunk) are damaged. As described previously for adults, an infant with an Erb's palsy maintains the arm (or arms) adducted, forearm extended and pronated, and wrist flexed (waiter's tip position). Another type of birth injury is Klumpke's palsy, with damage to the C8 and T1 nerve roots. Although this palsy can occur during a breech delivery with the arm hyper-abducted above the head, it most commonly occurs after a face-first delivery where the head is hyperextended. Infants with Klumpke's palsy are not able to grasp with the hand. Other types of birth brachial plexus injury include complete plexal injury and an Erb's *plus* palsy. An Erb's plus palsy is an injury involving C5, C6, *plus* C7.

Klumpke's palsy is the least common type of birth palsy. The prognosis of both Klumpke's palsy and complete brachial plexus palsy are both significantly worse than for Erb's palsy because the latter often recovers spontaneously in a matter of months.

Examining an infant is challenging. Neurological diagnosis of an obstetrical palsy relies greatly on observing the arm and hand position at rest, its lack of movement, and upper extremity asymmetry during play and crawling. Performing a series of examinations over time is important. Radiographs may be used to rule out fractures or a hemidiaphragm (phrenic palsy). Electrodiagnosis should be first performed 4 to 6 weeks after injury, and then on a serial basis (approximately every 3 months) when indicated to assess recovery. As the child grows, the examination becomes more structured, including various arm movements of functional importance.

Acute Brachial Plexitis (Parsonage–Turner Syndrome)

Acute brachial plexitis presents with marked shoulder pain that often radiates down the arm, up into the neck, or toward the scapula. Its onset is usually sudden and lasts for hours to a few weeks. This syndrome occurs more often in males and can affect any age group. A common position of comfort is the arm adducted and forearm flexed, the so-called adduction-flexion sign of acute brachial plexitis. Neck movement and Valsalva maneuvers do not exacerbate the pain. Cervical imaging helps rule out radiculopathy from a herniated disc.

Weakness is usually not present during the acute, painful phase of this syndrome; however, as the pain resolves, paralysis of certain brachial plexus innervated musculature occurs. The degree of eventual weakness often correlates with the severity of the initial pain. Although any, or all, upper extremity and shoulder girdle muscles may be involved, the most common muscles affected include the deltoid, supraspinatus, and infraspinatus. This syndrome may occur bilaterally, especially subclinically (i.e., seen only with electrodiagnostic testing). Sensory loss is classically absent or minimal during acute brachial plexitis, a finding that helps confirm the diagnosis. Because it is a benign and self-limiting process, approximately 90% of patients return to near normal in up to 3 years. The etiology of acute brachial plexitis is uncertain. About half of the patients report an antecedent, usually a viral illness, which points toward an inflammatory cause. Some patients report mild-to-moderate shoulder trauma or overuse as an instigating factor. Others may have recently undergone a surgical procedure. Electrophysiology is helpful for both diagnosis and prognosis.

- **A rare autosomal dominant form of acute brachial plexitis has been reported. These patients have repeated bouts of characteristic pain and weakness, often involving different nerves. Although these episodes often follow stressful events, including childbirth, strenuous exercise, and infection, the majority of cases have no identifiable cause. This hereditary disease can also affect children.**

Radiation-induced Brachial Plexopathy

Plexitis may occur following radiation treatment of regional cancers, usually breast cancer. Radiation damage can occur at any time after exposure (on average 5 years), and usually causes painless sensory and motor deficits in either the upper trunk or entire plexus; sole involvement of the lower trunk is uncommon. Horner's syndrome usually does not occur, and if it does, metastatic plexopathy or an apical lung metastasis should be investigated. Local radiation-induced skin changes are a common finding in these patients, although not universal. (See also the comments on radiation-induced plexitis in the lumbosacral plexus section.)

6

The Diagnostic Anatomy of the Sciatic Nerve

The sciatic nerve is the largest peripheral nerve in the body, and the lifeline to the lower extremities. It's sensory and motor function are so important that in the absence of proper medical care, severe, proximal sciatic nerve lesions can actually lead to limb amputation secondary to recurrent trauma and infection. Fortunately, with contemporary management of sciatic injuries this is not the rule; many patients recover some motor function, as well as enough protective sensation to ambulate and return to work.

Overall, the sciatic nerve mediates knee flexion and all motor function below the knee. The tibial half of the sciatic nerve controls plantar foot flexion, inversion, and the foot intrinsic muscles; the common peroneal portion controls foot dorsiflexion and eversion. Although both the tibial and common peroneal nerves carry sensation from large areas of the leg and foot, the sensation from the sole of the foot is by far the most important, which is carried by the tibial nerve.

♦ Anatomical Course

The Buttock

The sciatic nerve is the main product of the sacral plexus, being made up of fibers from the L4, L5, S1, S2, and S3 spinal nerves. After formation, the sciatic nerve exits the pelvis via the greater sciatic foramen inferior to the pyriformis muscle. The pyriformis muscle originates on the lateral intrapelvic surface of the sacrum and inserts on the most superior tip of the femur's greater trochanter. This muscle has a triangular shape, with its base on the sacrum and its apex on the trochanter.

After exiting the pelvis, the sciatic nerve runs distally toward the midline of the thigh, underneath the gluteus maximus, and over a bed of five successive muscles that run perpendicular to its course. In sequence, they are the following: superior gemelli, obturator internus, inferior gemelli, quadratus femoris, and the adductor magnus. The sciatic nerve remains posterior (dorsal) to the adductor magnus as it courses down the thigh (**Fig. 6–1**). The first three muscles (superior gemelli, obturator internus, and inferior gemelli) form a group and attach to the greater trochanter. The quadratus femoris inserts into the lesser trochanter; the adductor magnus has a long insertion on the shaft of the femur.

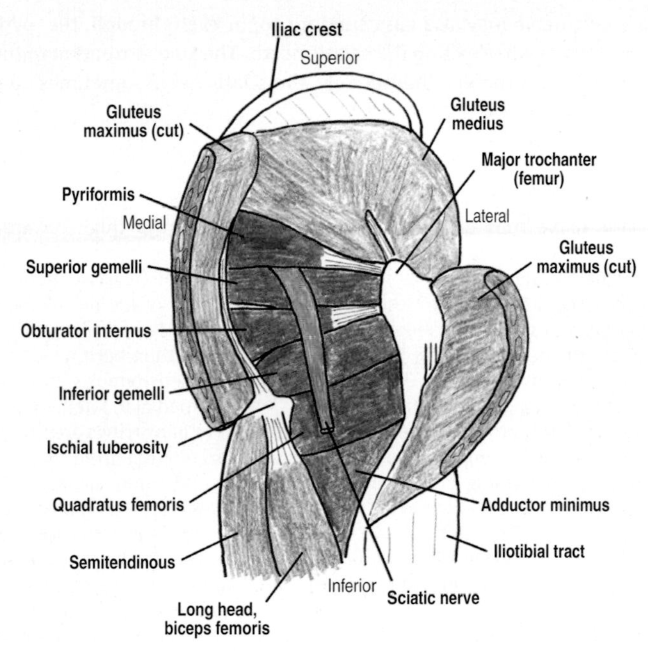

Figure 6–1 The muscular anatomy of the piriformis and deep buttock muscles. After formation, the sciatic nerve exits the pelvis via the greater sciatic foramen inferior to the pyriformis muscle. After leaving the pelvis, the sciatic nerve then runs distally toward the midline of the thigh, underneath the gluteus maximus and over a bed of five successive muscles that run perpendicular to its course.

The sciatic nerve is actually two nerves, the tibial and common peroneal, which are joined by a common epineurium from the pelvis to the lower third of the thigh where these two components separate. The tibial nerve is medial and larger, being composed of fibers from L4 through S3. The common peroneal nerve is lateral and smaller, and is composed of fibers from fewer spinal nerves, specifically L4-S2, with a large contribution from the lumbosacral trunk. Before forming the sciatic nerve, the ventral rami of these spinal nerves split into anterior and posterior divisions, with the tibial nerve being composed of the anterior divisions and the common peroneal by the posterior divisions. This orientation is opposite than expected because the tibial nerve innervates posterior compartment muscles, whereas the common peroneal nerve innervates anterior compartment ones. The sciatic nerve is protected by the large gluteus maximus, as well as by the ischial tuberosity when one sits.

Also exiting the pelvis through the greater sciatic notch under the pyriformis muscle, but medial to the sciatic nerve, are the posterior cutaneous nerve to the thigh (the lesser sciatic nerve), the inferior gluteal nerve and vessels, and most medially, the pudendal nerve and vessels. The superior gluteal nerve exits the greater sciatic foramen superior to the pyriformis. These nerves are discussed in the lumbosacral plexus section.

♦ The sciatic nerve may also pass superior to, or even through, the pyriformis muscle when exiting the sciatic notch. The S3 contribution to the sciatic nerve is variable. Alternatively, the sciatic nerve sometimes contains fibers from S4.

The Thigh and Knee

The sciatic nerve runs down the midline of the posterior thigh toward the popliteal fossa. It runs superficial, or dorsal, to the adductor magnus, but underneath the hamstring muscles. There are four hamstring muscles, two medial and two lateral. The lateral pair are the long and short heads of the biceps femoris. The long head of the biceps femoris originates from the ischial tuberosity; the short head originates from the shaft of the femur. Together, both heads insert distally into the fibular head. The long head of the biceps femoris crosses the midline of the thigh, similar to the arm of an "X," from medial to lateral. The long head is superficial to the short head. The medial pair of hamstrings are the semitendinous and semimembranous muscles, both originating from the ischial tuberosity and remaining medial along the thigh to insert into the lateral tibia, along with the sartorius and gracilis tendons. The semitendinous is more superficial and medial. The sciatic nerve runs deep to the hamstrings, remaining mostly deep to the long head of the biceps femoris as this muscle runs medial to lateral. The sciatic nerve bifurcates into the tibial and common peroneal nerves approximately two thirds of the way down the thigh. Distally, like the archway of a door, both the medial and lateral groups of hamstrings part away from midline to expose the popliteal fossa.

The larger and more-medial tibial nerve (anterior divisions of L4 to S3) continues down the thigh and into the popliteal fossa while remaining midline. In the distal thigh, the tibial nerve joins the popliteal artery and vein. These vessels are the distal continuations of the femoral artery and vein, and enter the posterior compartment of the thigh by passing medial to the femur via the adductor hiatus. Viewing the popliteal fossa from posterior, the tibial nerve lies lateral to the popliteal vessels **(Fig. 6–2).** This neurovascular bundle runs deep into the leg (defined as the lower extremity between the knee and the ankle) by passing under the gastrocnemius and soleus muscles. Underneath these proximal calf muscles, the tibial nerve runs over or dorsal to the popliteal muscle, which creates the floor of the popliteal fossa by running transversely from the upper medial aspect of the tibia to the lower lateral femur.

Prior to entering the leg, the tibial nerve branches to the *medial sural cutaneous nerve*. This branch runs superficially along the midline between the two heads of the gastrocnemius muscle, eventually piercing the subcutaneous fascia just distal to this muscle. Upon piercing the fascia, the medial sural cutaneous nerve merges with the *lateral sural cutaneous nerve* (from the common peroneal nerve) to form the proper *sural nerve*. The sural nerve runs down the posterior leg, behind the lateral malleolus, and into the dorsolateral foot.

The common peroneal nerve (posterior divisions of L4-S2) runs obliquely from the apex of the popliteal fossa to the posterior fibular head (**Fig. 6–2**). In doing so, this nerve skirts along the medial margin of the biceps femoris muscle. In this region, the common peroneal nerve gives off two sensory branches, the lateral sural cutaneous (mentioned previously), which merges with the medial sural cutaneous (from the tibial nerve), and the *lateral cutaneous nerve to the calf*. Following these two branches, the common peroneal nerve passes lateral to the very proximal fibular shaft, underneath the peroneus longus muscle.

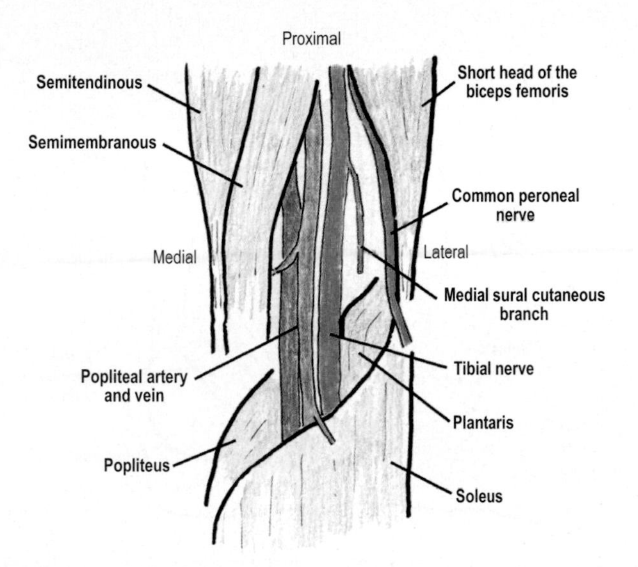

Figure 6–2 Popliteal fossa anatomy. Viewing the popliteal fossa from posterior, the tibial nerve lies lateral to the popliteal artery and vein. The common peroneal nerve skirts along the medial margin of the biceps femoris muscle, from the apex of the popliteal fossa to the fibular head.

The sural nerve is usually made up of both medial and lateral sural cutaneous nerves; however, in some patients the sural nerve is derived from only one of these two nerves, usually the medial one.

The Tibial Nerve

The Leg

The tibial nerve runs down the leg in a straight line from the middle of the popliteal fossa, to just posterior to the medial malleolus. This nerve runs deep to the gastrocnemius and soleus muscles, but remains superficial (dorsal) to the deep posterior compartment muscles. In the proximal leg, the tibial nerve runs on, or dorsal to, the tibialis posterior muscle. In the distal leg it runs in a cleft between the flexor digitorum longus medially, and the flexor hallucis longus laterally. The popliteal artery and vein continue with the tibial nerve in the leg, but are renamed the posterior tibial artery and vein. These vessels run on the nerve's medial aspect, first over the tibialis posterior, then over the flexor digitorum longus.

Posterior to the medial malleolus, the tibial nerve enters the foot by running deep to the flexor retinaculum (lacinate ligament). The flexor retinaculum is a thin ligament that bridges the medial malleolus to the calcaneus, under which passes not only the tibial nerve, but also the posterior tibial artery and veins, and from anterior to posterior, the tendons of the tibialis posterior, flexor digitorum longus, and flexor hallucis longus. This subligamentous, anatomic passage into the foot is called the *tarsal tunnel* (**Fig. 6–3**).

Within, or just proximal, to the tarsal tunnel, the tibial nerve bifurcates into the medial and lateral plantar nerves. The tibial nerve also gives a sensory branch to the medial half of the heel just before, or from within, the tarsal tunnel. This branch is called the *medial calcaneal nerve.*

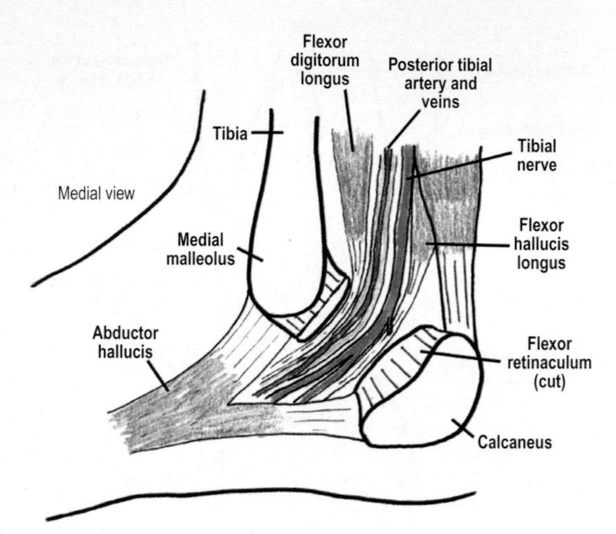

Figure 6–3 The tarsal tunnel. Posterior to the medial malleolus, the tibial nerve enters the foot by running deep to the flexor retinaculum. The flexor retinaculum is a ligamentous band from the medial malleolus to the calcaneus, under which passes not only the tibial nerve, but also the posterior tibial artery, veins, and multiple tendons.

The Foot

The medial plantar nerve is the larger of the two terminal divisions of the tibial nerve, and as its name implies, courses through the medial plantar region (**Fig. 6–4**). The medial plantar nerve runs between the abductor hallucis and the flexor digitorum brevis, the latter muscle being located in the midline of the sole. As the medial plantar nerve courses down the foot, it progressively bifurcates into digital nerves for the first three and a half toes. Sensory branches to the sole originate quite proximal, just after the medial plantar nerve enters the sole of the foot.

After traversing the tarsal tunnel, the lateral plantar nerve passes across the sole of the foot, deep to the flexor digitorum brevis. Once lateral, it runs anteriorly between the quadratus plantae medially and the abductor digiti minimi pedis laterally. The lateral plantar nerve divides into a superficial sensory and deep motor branch, analogous to the ulnar nerve in the hand. The superficial branch becomes subcutaneous and the deep branch remains deep to innervate the intrinsic foot musculature.

The Common Peroneal Nerve

The Deep Branch

The common peroneal nerve passes around the lateral aspect of the upper fibula, just distal to the fibular head, underneath the posterior fibrous edge of the peroneus longus muscle. Two ligamentous bands in this region form the so-called fibular tunnel: the peroneus longus muscle aponeurosis (deep) and an aponeurosis connecting the soleus and peroneal fascia (superficial). Under the peroneus longus, the common peroneal nerve bifurcates into a superficial and deep branch.

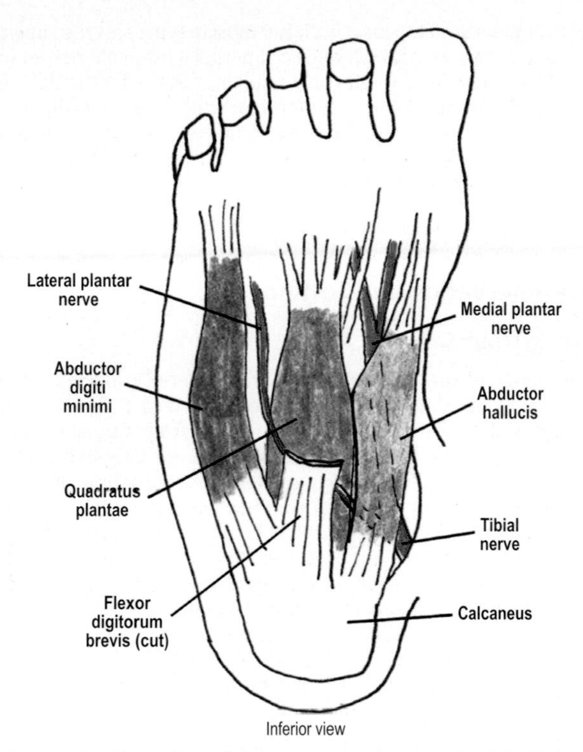

Figure 6–4 Muscle relationships of the plantar nerves in the sole of the foot. The medial plantar nerve runs between the abductor hallucis and the flexor digitorum brevls, the latter muscle being located in the midline of the sole. The lateral plantar nerve passes across the sole of the foot, deep to the flexor digitorum brevis. Once lateral, it runs anteriorly between the quadratus plantae medially and the abductor digiti minimi pedis laterally.

Anterior to the fibula, the deep peroneal nerve dives deep to the extensor digitorum longus muscle, where it joins the tibialis anterior artery to travel down the leg. This neurovascular bundle runs between the extensor digitorum longus anteriorly and the intermuscular septum/lateral tibia posteriorly. In the more distal aspect of the leg, the deep peroneal nerve shifts a little toward the midline, where it runs on the tibia under the tibialis anterior muscle. The deep peroneal nerve passes onto the dorsal aspect of the foot by running under two extensor retinaculums (superior and inferior), a confined anatomical space known as the *anterior tarsal tunnel.* Once on the dorsum of the foot, the deep peroneal nerve divides into medial and lateral branches. The medial branch passes distally with the dorsalis pedis artery, eventually terminating as a sensory branch to the first web space. The lateral branch innervates the extensor digitorum brevis.

The Superficial Branch

The superficial branch of the common peroneal nerve turns distally after passing around the fibula to run under the peroneus longus. It, however, remains superficial to the extensor digitorum longus. This latter muscle separates the superficial and deep branches of the peroneal nerve. The superficial branch emerges in the distal half of the leg, lateral to the formed tendon of the peroneus longus muscle and still superficial to the extensor digitorum longus. This nerve divides into two sensory branches proximal to the extensor retinaculum. Both of these branches run superficial to the extensor retinaculum; they are called the *medial and intermediate, dorsal cutaneous nerves of the foot.*

♦ Motor Innervation and Testing

The Buttock/Thigh Group

Immediately after exiting the pelvis, the sciatic nerve provides two common motor branches to innervate the hamstring muscles (**Fig. 6–5**). One branch originates from the tibial division; the second comes from the common peroneal division. These hamstring branches pass distally with the sciatic nerve in the buttock region. The sciatic nerve also gives supplementary branches to the hamstring muscles as it passes next to them in the more distal thigh, however, loss of these smaller branches, in general, may not be noticed clinically when the larger, proximal hamstring branches are preserved. Considering the proximal origin of the main hamstring branches, a sciatic nerve injury involving the hamstring muscles would have to be very proximal (e.g., the buttock region).

The tibial portion of the sciatic nerve innervates the medial hamstrings (the *semitendinous* and *semimembranous*), as well as the *long head of the biceps femoris*. The *short head of the biceps femoris* is the only hamstring innervated by

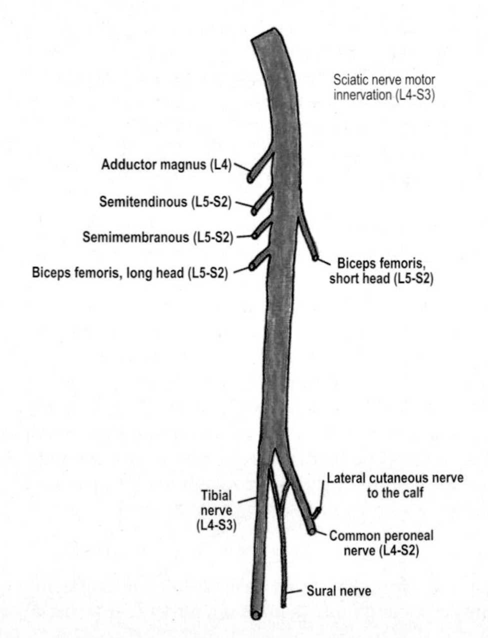

Figure 6–5 Motor innervation from the sciatic (schematic) nerve in the buttock and thigh.

the more lateral common peroneal portion of the sciatic nerve. The hamstrings (L5-S2) are tested with the patient seated, instructing him or her to flex the leg against resistance. The examiner should simultaneously palpate the hamstring tendons in the proximal popliteal fossa (**Fig. 6–6**). The hamstrings may also be tested with the patient prone. An isolated lesion affecting only the tibial half of the sciatic nerve spares the peroneal innervated short head of the biceps femoris. In this situation, a portion of the lateral hamstrings will continue to function, and its tendon can be palpated during thigh flexion.

The tibial portion of the sciatic nerve also innervates the ischial half of the *adductor magnus* (L4 of L2-L4). Test this muscle, along with the other thigh

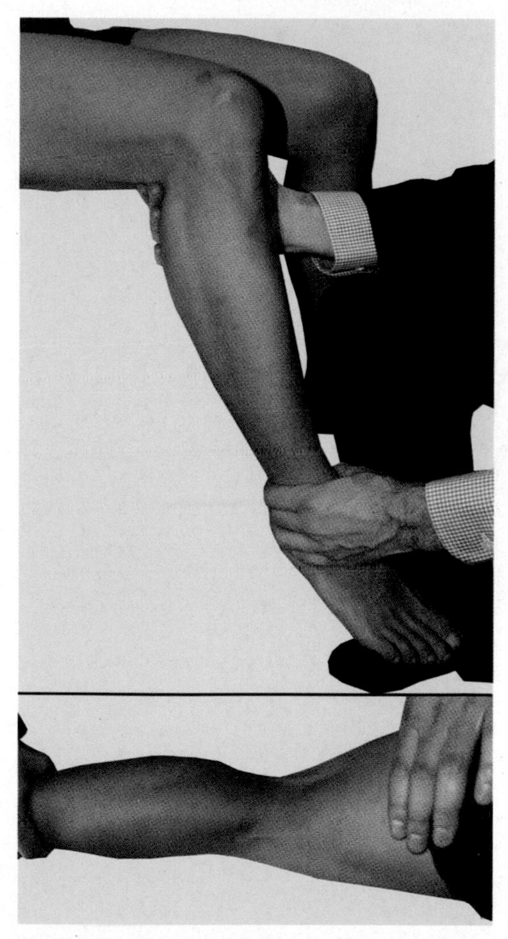

Figure 6–6 Hamstring (L5-S2) assessment: The hamstrings are tested with the patient seated. Instruct the patient to flex at the knee against resistance. The examiner should simultaneously palpate the hamstring tendons in the proximal popliteal fossa. The hamstrings may also be tested with the patient prone (lower image).

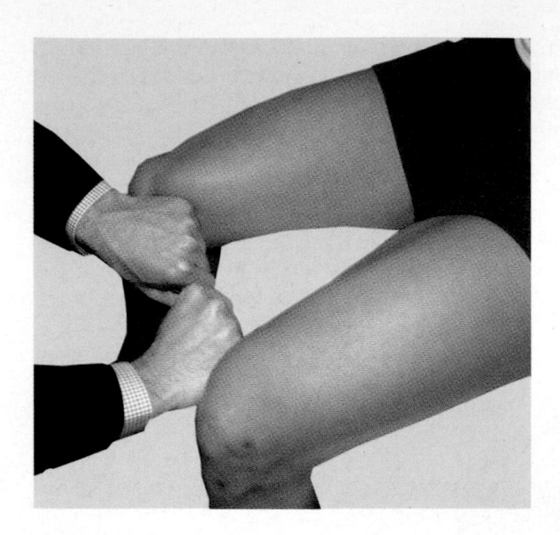

Figure 6–7 Thigh adduction (L2-L4) assessment: Test thigh adduction by having the patient bring the knees together against resistance, with the patient either seated or supine. (The sciatic nerve provides only L4 contribution; L2 and L3 contribution is carried by the obturator nerve.)

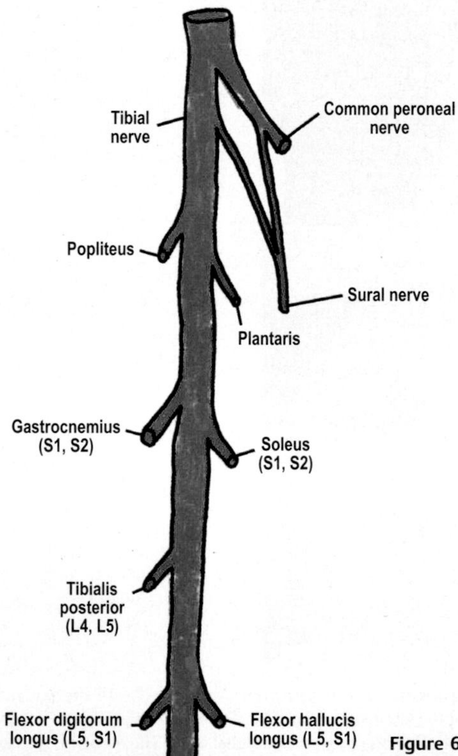

Figure 6–8 Motor innervation from the tibial nerve in the leg (L4–S2).

adductors (innervated by the obturator nerve), by having the patient bring the knees together under resistance, either seated (**Fig. 6–7**) or supine.

The Leg

The Tibial Nerve Group

The tibial nerve innervates the posterior compartment muscles of the leg, which control plantar flexion, foot inversion, and toe flexion (**Fig. 6–8**). Prior to passing deep to the *gastrocnemius* and *soleus* (S1, S2), the tibial nerve sends branches to these muscles. Therefore, damage to the tibial nerve deep to these muscles would spare their innervation. Although both the gastrocnemius (medial and lateral heads) and soleus muscles insert into the calcaneus, they have different origins. The gastrocnemius originates from the distal femur and therefore produces plantar flexion with the knee straight. In contrast, the soleus originates from the tibia and therefore can mediate plantar flexion with the knee straight or bent. Because the gastrocnemius is so powerful with the knee straight, soleus-mediated plantar flexion is only dominant when the knee is flexed. With the patient sitting, the gastrocnemius heads can be tested by extending the leg at the knee and having the patient plantar flex the foot against resistance ("pushing down on the gas pedal")(**Fig. 6–9**). Gastrocnemius contraction should be palpated. The soleus is tested in near-isolation (gastrocnemius function can never be eliminated) by instructing the patient to go up on his or her toes while seated with the knees flexed (**Fig. 6–10**). To observe subtle plantar flexion weakness, the patient should attempt to stand on his or her toes, one foot at a time.

Immediately deep to the soleus, the tibial nerve innervates the *tibialis posterior* (L4, L5). This muscle is the prime inverter of the foot, with its tendon inserting into the tarsal bones both on the medial aspect of the foot, as well as on the lateral aspect, that is after passing underneath the foot. Test the tibialis posterior by having the patient invert the foot against resistance (**Fig. 6–11**). Toes flexors should remain relaxed to avoid substitution. Alternatively, the patient can place the soles of his or her feet together while in a sitting position.

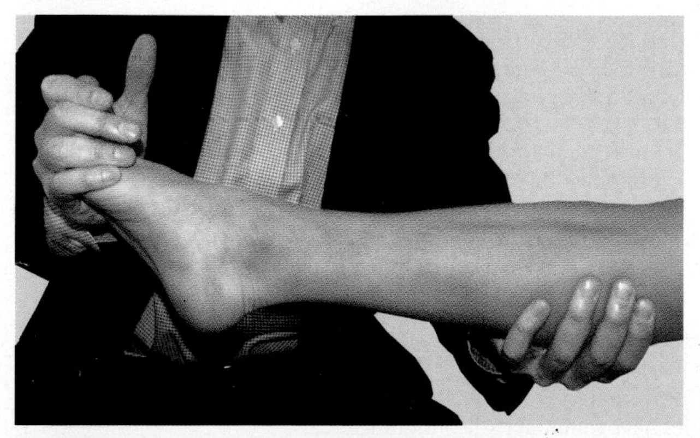

Figure 6–9 Gastrocnemius (S1, S2) assessment: With the patient sitting, the gastrocnemius heads are tested by having the patient plantar flex the foot against resistance with the knee straight. The examiner's other hand stabilizes the leg and palpates gastrocnemius contraction. To observe subtle plantar flexion weakness, the patient should attempt to stand on his or her toes, one foot at a time, or even walk on the toes.

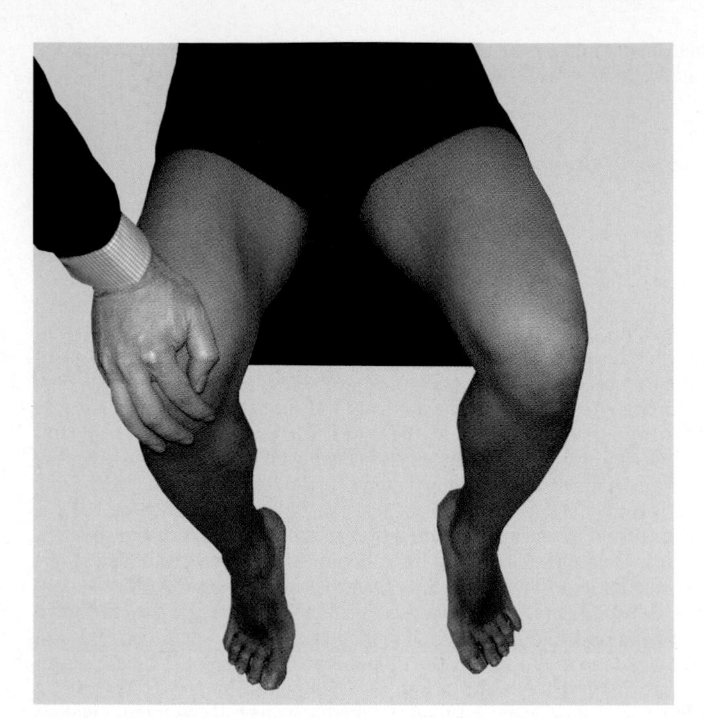

Figure 6–10 Soleus (S1, S2) assessment: The soleus is tested in near-isolation by instructing the patient to go up on his or her toes while seated, with resistance placed on the knee tops.

In the posterior leg compartment, the tibial nerve also innervates the *flexor digitorum longus* and *flexor hallucis longus* (L5, S1). Tendons from these muscles insert into the most distal phalanges of the toes, and thereby mediate flexion in all the joints they cross. To assess these muscles (along with the similar acting flexor digitorum brevis), one instructs the patient to curl the toes against resistance. Resistance is applied by grasping the foot with both hands, using the fingers to hold the dorsum of the foot while both thumbs force the toes back into extension (**Fig. 6–12**). The flexor hallucis longus acts on the great toe while the flexor digitorum longus inserts into the rest.

- **Together, the long toe flexors, peroneus muscles, and tibialis posterior can substitute for plantar flexion. This substitution, however, mostly flexes the forefoot, not necessarily the ankle. In the distal popliteal fossa, the tibial nerve innervates the *popliteus* and *plantaris* muscles. These two muscles have minimal clinical significance.**

The Deep Peroneal Nerve Group

The deep peroneal nerve innervates all anterior compartment leg muscles, excluding the peroneus longus and brevis, which are innervated by the superficial peroneal

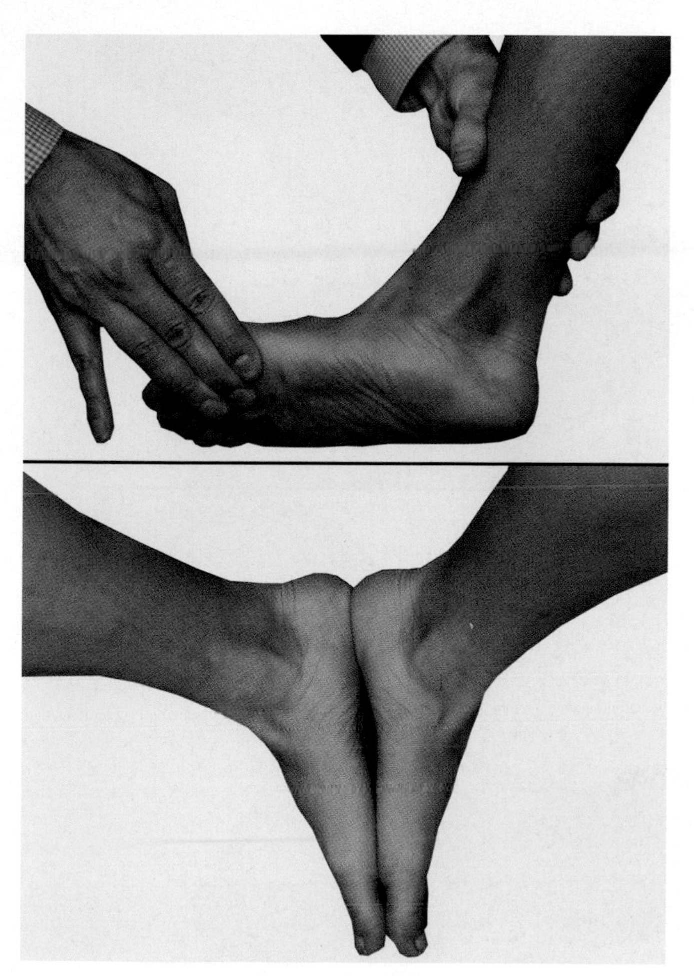

Figure 6–11 Tibialis posterior (L4, L5) assessment: The tibialis posterior is tested with the patient inverting the foot against resistance. Toes flexors should remain relaxed to avoid substitution. Alternatively, the patient can place the soles of the feet together while in a sitting position (lower image).

nerve (**Fig. 6–13**). Immediately after passing deep to the extensor digitorum longus, the deep peroneal nerve gives a motor branch to the *tibialis anterior* (L4-S1), which is the prime dorsiflexor of the foot. Weakness of the tibialis anterior, with sparing of the peroneus muscles, indicates an injury to the deep peroneal nerve near its origin at the fibula. Contraction of the tibialis anterior can be seen and palpated during muscle testing (**Fig. 6–14**). The toes should remain relaxed, because contraction of the toes extensors can substitute for foot dorsiflexion.

The *deep peroneal nerve innervates the extensor digitorum longus* (L5, S1) and *extensor hallucis longus* (L5). Tendons from these muscles insert into the distal

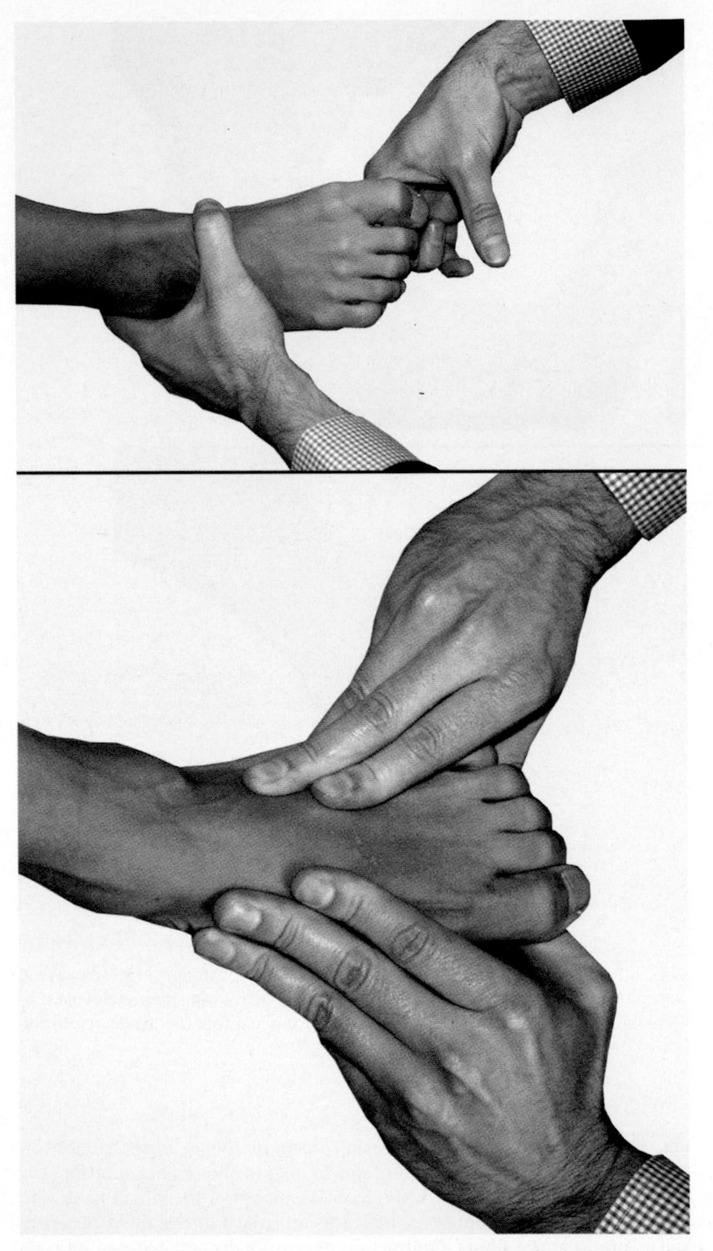

Figure 6–12 Flexors digitorum longus, flexor hallucis longus (both L5, S1), and flexor digitorum brevis (S1, S2) assessment: To assess toe flexion, instruct the patient to curl the toes against resistance. Alternatively, resistance can be applied by grasping the foot with both hands, using the fingers to hold the dorsum of the foot and both thumbs to force the toes back into extension (lower image).

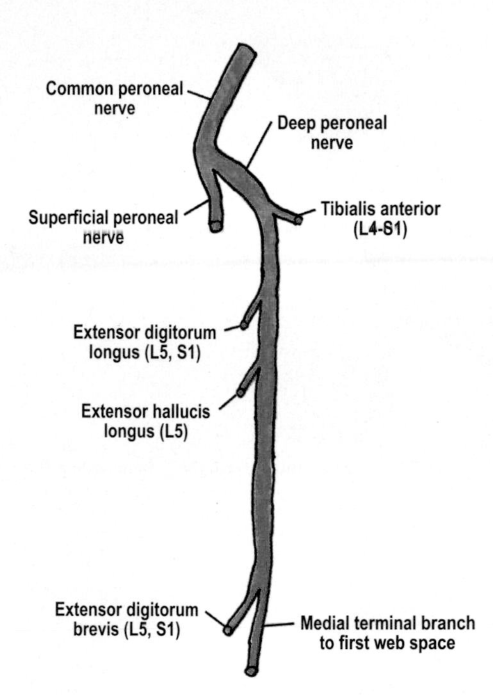

Figure 6–13 Motor innervation from the deep peroneal nerve (L4–S1).

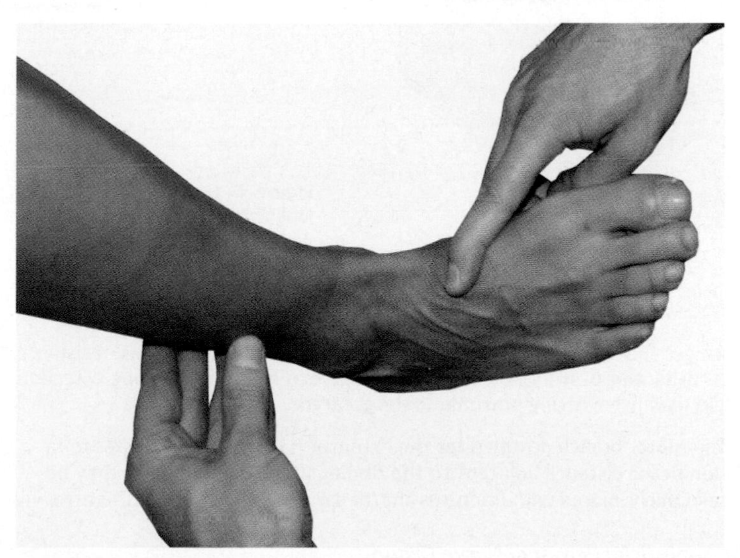

Figure 6–14 Tibialis anterior (L4-S1) assessment: Contraction of this muscle can be seen during foot dorsiflexion. The toes should remain relaxed because the toe extensors may substitute for foot dorsiflexion.

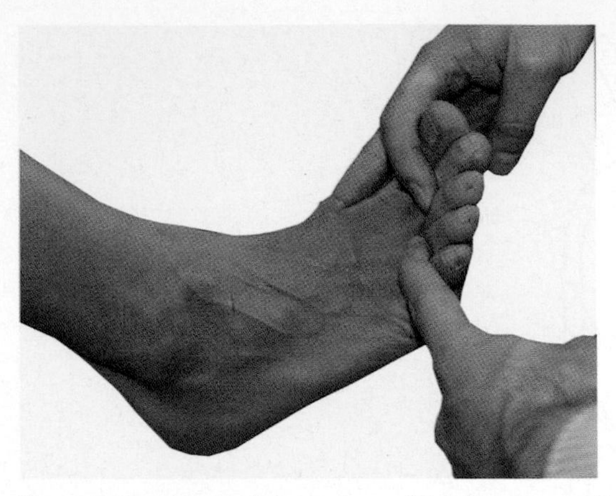

Figure 6–15 Extensor digitorum longus (L5, S1) assessment: Have the patient extend the toes, with or without resistance.

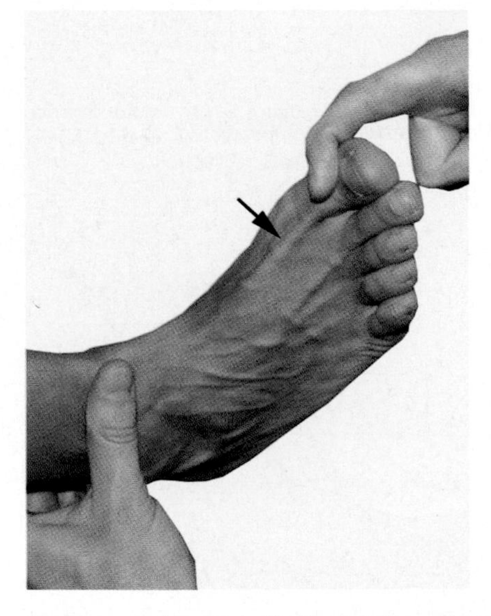

Figure 6–16 Extensor hallucis longus (L5) assessment: Have the patient extend the great toe against resistance. The tendon (arrow) should readily bowstring proximal to the great toe upon contraction.

phalanges and are tested by having the patient extend the toes against resistance (**Figs. 6–15 and 6–16**). Upon contraction, the extensor hallucis longus tendon should readily bowstring proximal to the great toe.

- **The motor branch destined for the extensor hallucis longus passes for a significant distance adjacent to the fibular shaft, and therefore may be selectively injured with fractures and/or surgical procedures in this area.**

The Superficial Peroneal Nerve Group

The superficial peroneal nerve mediates foot eversion by innervating the *peroneus longus and brevis* (L5, S1) in the lateral aspect (compartment) of the leg

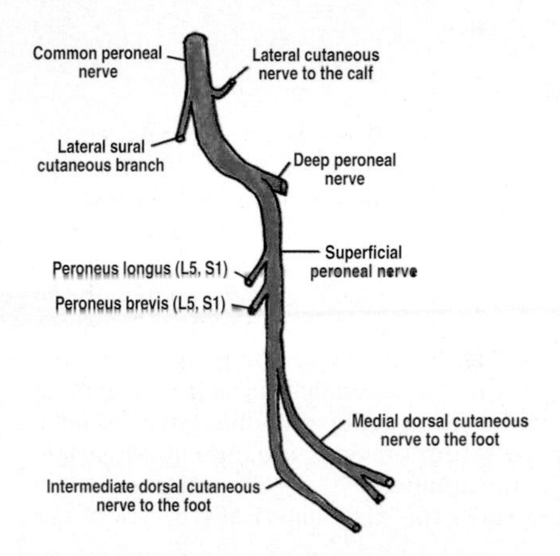

Figure 6–17 Motor innervation of the superficial peroneal nerve (L5–S1).

(**Fig. 6–17**). Both of these muscles originate from the fibula, and insert into the foot after passing around the posterior aspect of the lateral malleolus. The peroneus brevis simply inserts into the undersurface of the fifth metatarsal. The peroneus longus, however, mirroring the tibialis posterior, loops around the undersurface of the foot to insert into the proximal portion of the first metatarsal. The peroneus muscles are evaluated by having the patient evert the foot against resistance (**Fig. 6–18**). Contraction of these muscles can be observed and palpated. The peroneus brevis tendon bowstrings the skin between the lateral malleolus and its insertion into the fifth metatarsal head.

- **Although not present in most people, a lateral extension of the extensor digitorum longus, called the *peroneus tertius*, may be present. This muscle is innervated by the *superficial* peroneal nerve (not the deep peroneal nerve that innervates the extensor digitorum longus), and inserts into the fifth metatarsal, mediating "extension" of the foot's lateral aspect.**

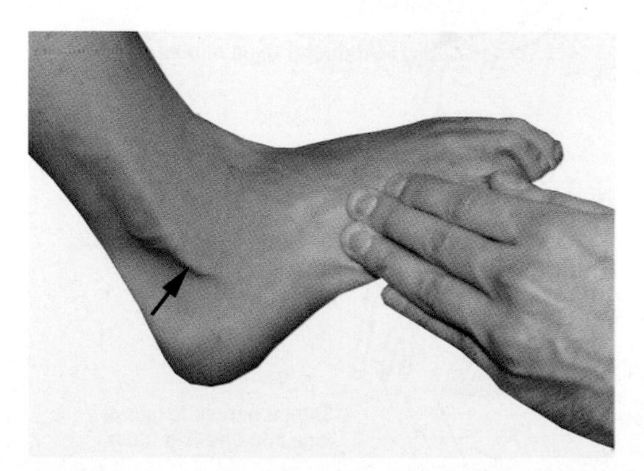

Figure 6–18 Peroneus longus and brevis (L5, S1) assessment: The peroneus muscles are evaluated by having the patient evert the foot against resistance. Contraction of these muscles can be observed and palpated. The tendon (arrow) of the peroneus brevis can be observed bowstringing the skin between the lateral malleolus and its insertion into the fifth metatarsal head.

The Foot

The Medial Plantar Nerve Group

Upon passing between the *abductor hallucis* and *flexor digitorum brevis* (S1, S2), the medial plantar nerve innervates these two muscles (**Fig. 6–19**). The tendons of the flexor digitorum brevis insert into the proximal phalanges of the second through fifth toes, and mediate flexion at the metatarsal–phalangeal joints. More distally, the medial plantar nerve also innervates the *flexor hallucis brevis* (S1, S2), which likewise flexes the metatarsal–phalangeal joint of the great toe. These muscles are difficult to isolate on examination; however, composite toe flexion can be tested (**Fig. 6–20**). When the patient curls the arch of the foot medially, the abductor hallucis usually contracts well enough to be tested. When denervated, atrophy of the abductor hallucis may be seen. In contrast, wasting of the flexor digitorum brevis is usually not noticeable because of the thick sole and plantar aponeurosis covering it. The medial plantar nerve also commonly innervates the *first lumbrical* (L5, S1) of the foot.

The Lateral Plantar Nerve Group

The lateral plantar nerve and its deep branch innervate most of the intrinsic muscles of the foot, analogous to the ulnar nerve in the hand **(Fig. 6–19).** These muscles include the *quadratus plantae*, *abductor digiti minimi pedis*, *second to fourth lumbricals* all the *dorsal interossei*, and both heads of the *adductor hallucis* (all via S1-S3). Foot intrinsic muscles innervated by other

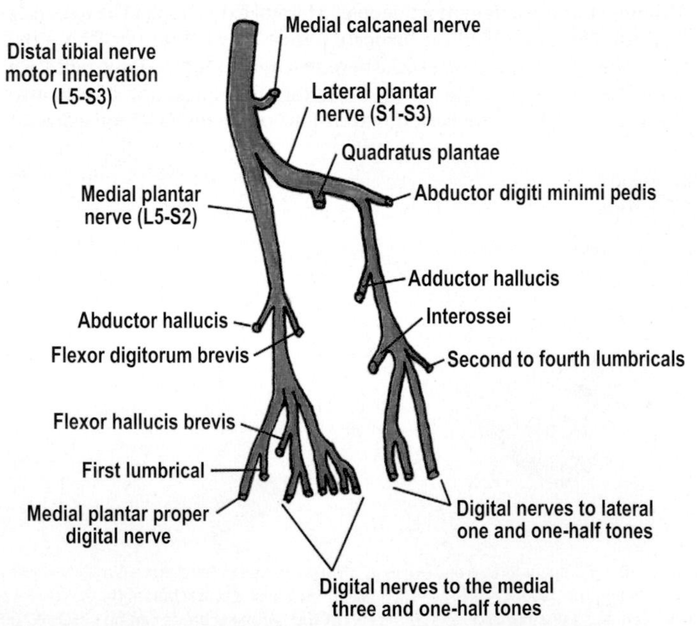

Figure 6–19 Motor innervation from the plantar nerves in the sole of the foot.

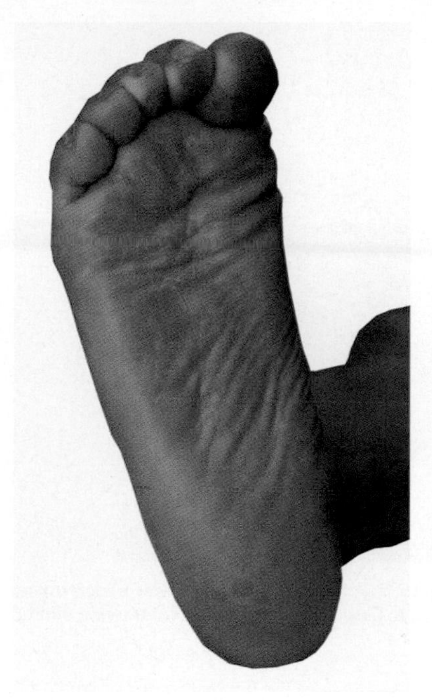

Figure 6–20 Cupping of the sole (S1-S3): Grossly assess intrinsic motor function by instructing the patient to "cup" the foot. Alternatively, you can have him or her spread the toes; however, some patients with normal motor function are not able to do this. Action of the individual foot intrinsic muscles cannot be easily isolated on physical examination.

nerves include the abductor hallucis, flexor digitorum brevis, and flexor hallucis brevis (medial plantar nerve), as well as two muscles on the dorsum of the foot, the extensors digitorum and hallucis brevis (deep peroneal nerve, see below). One may grossly assess intrinsic motor function by instructing the patient to "cup" the foot (**Fig. 6–20**). Action of the individual foot intrinsic muscles cannot be readily isolated on physical examination. Chronic, severe intrinsic foot muscle weakness can cause clawing of the toes.

The Deep Peroneal Nerve Group

The lateral terminal branch of the deep peroneal nerve in the dorsum of the foot innervates the *extensor digitorum brevis* (L5, S1). This muscle extends the toes at the metatarsal-phalangeal joint, a movement that is hard to isolate from the extensors digitorum and hallucis longus. The best way to determine paralysis of the extensor digitorum brevis is to observe and palpate its contraction during composite toe extension (**Fig. 6–21**).

♦ The Accessory Peroneal Nerve

The accessory peroneal nerve is a distal branch of the superficial peroneal nerve that is present in approximately 20% of people. This branch carries motor innervation to the extensor digitorum brevis, a muscle that is usually controlled by the

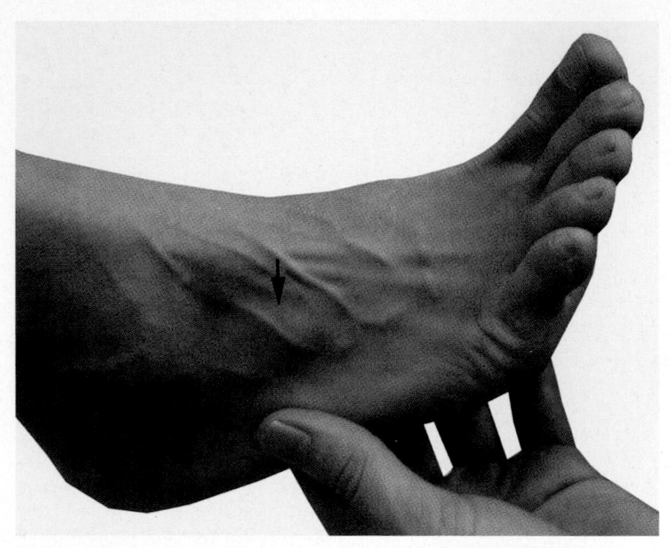

Figure 6–21 Extensor digitorum brevis (L5, S1) assessment: The best way to determine paralysis of the extensor digitorum brevis is to observe and palpate its contraction during toe extension (arrow).

deep peroneal nerve. When evaluating electrophysiological and clinical examination results, one should keep this potential transfer of motor innervation in mind when localizing the lesion.

- **The accessory peroneal nerve may occasionally branch from the deep peroneal nerve.**

♦ Sensory Innervation

The *sural nerve* provides sensory coverage to the lower lateral leg, some lateral heel and ankle, and the dorsolateral aspect of the foot, especially its lateral margin (**Fig. 6–22**). Because of overlap in sensory coverage of the leg and foot, damage to the sural nerve (e.g., following an excisional biopsy) usually only manifests as numbness along the lateral border of the foot. With time, however, this area of numbness shrinks as the neighboring sensory nerves branch to cover the loss. The sural nerve is composed of two communicating branches, one from the tibial nerve and the other from the common peroneal nerve. The tibial nerve gives the medial sural cutaneous nerve in the popliteal fossa, whose distal continuation becomes the sural nerve proper. The common peroneal nerve in the popliteal fossa yields two sensory branches, the lateral sural cutaneous and lateral cutaneous nerve to the calf. The first of which, as the name implies, carries fibers destined for the sural nerve. The medial and lateral sural cutaneous nerves merge just below the two heads of the gastrocnemius muscle either before or after the medial sural cutaneous nerve pierces the fascia to become subcutaneous.

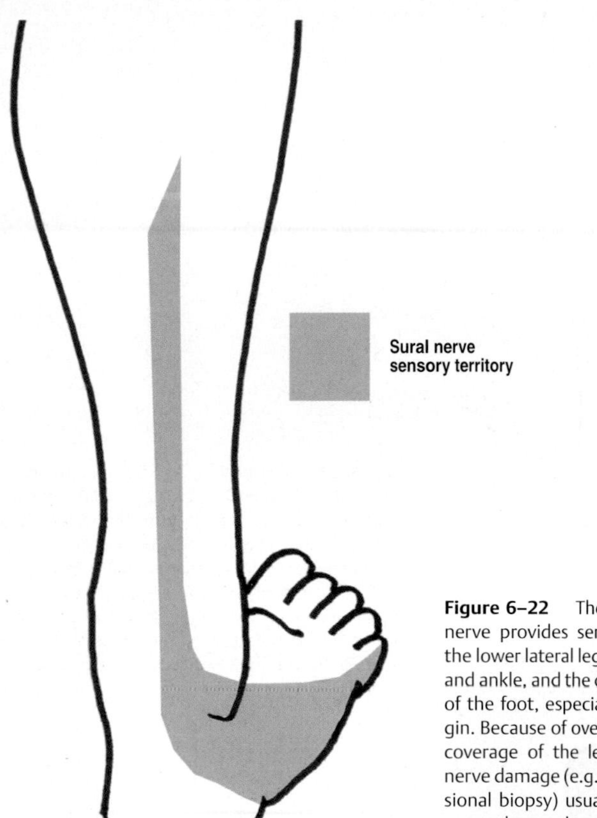

Figure 6–22 The Sural nerve. This nerve provides sensory coverage to the lower lateral leg, some lateral heel and ankle, and the dorsolateral aspect of the foot, especially its lateral margin. Because of overlap in the sensory coverage of the leg and foot, sural nerve damage (e.g., following an excisional biopsy) usually only manifests as numbness along the lateral border of the foot.

The *lateral cutaneous nerve to the calf* provides sensory coverage of the lateral knee and calf (i.e., the upper lateral aspect of the leg). The remaining lower lateral portion of the leg is covered by either the sural nerve, the lateral sural cutaneous branch, or cutaneous branches off the superficial peroneal nerve. The lateral cutaneous nerve to the calf does not have a consistent autonomous region to test.

Together, the deep and superficial peroneal nerves provide sensation to the dorsum of the foot and anterolateral shin (**Fig. 6–23**). The *superficial peroneal nerve* carries the majority of this sensation, except for a small area of skin centered on the web space between the first and second toes, which the *deep peroneal nerve* covers.

The tibial division of the sciatic nerve carries the most important sensation of the lower extremity, that for the sole of the foot (**Fig. 6–24**). With numbness in the sole of the foot, minor trauma, or unrecognized, persistent pressure, may cause ulcers, infection, and even amputation. Furthermore, dysesthesias in this region may prevent ambulation and be very problematic. The tibial nerve's coverage of the foot's plantar aspect is divided into three zones. The *medial calcaneal nerve* exits the tibial nerve just prior, or within, the tarsal tunnel, and innervates

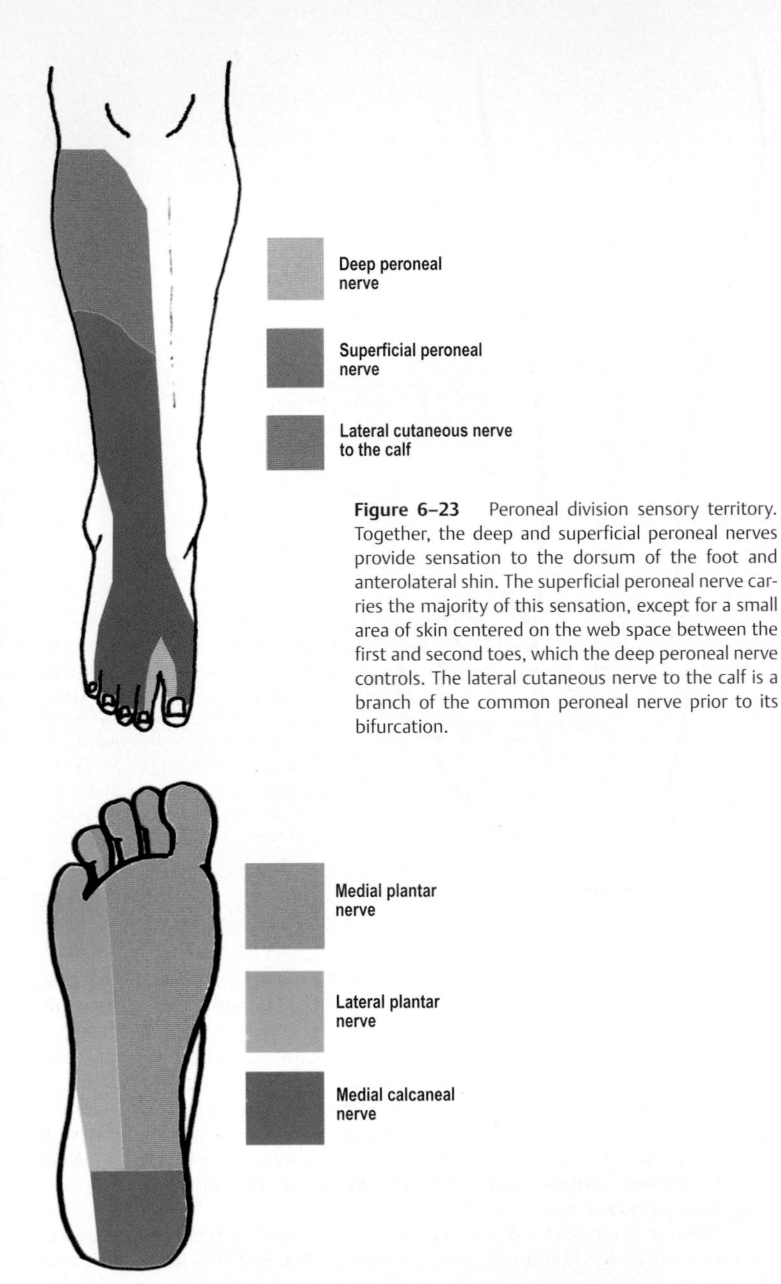

Figure 6–23 Peroneal division sensory territory. Together, the deep and superficial peroneal nerves provide sensation to the dorsum of the foot and anterolateral shin. The superficial peroneal nerve carries the majority of this sensation, except for a small area of skin centered on the web space between the first and second toes, which the deep peroneal nerve controls. The lateral cutaneous nerve to the calf is a branch of the common peroneal nerve prior to its bifurcation.

Figure 6–24 Tibial division sensory territory. Three branches from the tibial nerve cover the foot's plantar aspect. The medial calcaneal nerve exits the tibial nerve just prior, or within, the tarsal tunnel, and innervates the medial half of the heel. The medial and lateral plantar nerves provide sensory branches to the medial and lateral sole, respectively.

the medial half of the heel. The *medial and lateral plantar nerves* provide sensory branches to the medial and lateral sole, respectively. The medial plantar nerve covers a bit more area, including the first three and one-half toes, and the lateral plantar nerve covers the lateral one and a half toes. The plantar nerve's sensory coverage includes the nails and the skin surrounding the nails on the toes' dorsal surfaces. A branch of the sural nerve covers sensation on the lateral heel, although this may be inconsistent.

♦ Clinical Findings and Syndromes

The Buttock

Trauma, Fractures, and Injections

A complete sciatic nerve lesion is a severe deficit. Sensation to the lateral aspect of the leg and nearly all of the foot is lost. The only sensation remaining in the foot is near the medial malleolus, which is carried by the saphenous nerve. Sensory loss, as mentioned earlier in this chapter, is probably the most dangerous aspect of a severe sciatic nerve palsy. Proper shoes and daily foot checks by the patient are mandatory until enough protective sensation of the sole and foot is recovered. Regarding motor control, all foot and ankle movements are lost, which may preclude useful ambulation without the use of orthotics. Loss of leg flexion at the knee can also occur for complete, proximal sciatic nerve palsies. Hamstring weakness, however, is uncommon because the major branches to these muscles originate from the sciatic nerve quite proximally, sometimes at or within the sciatic notch. For this reason, most sciatic nerve palsies actually spare leg flexion at the knee.

Care must be taken when attempting to differentiate a sciatic nerve injury from an S1 radiculopathy or sacral plexus injury. Making this differentiation is often not possible using only the neurological examination. An S1 radiculopathy frequently involves the gluteal nerves, whereas a sciatic nerve palsy would not. However, depending on the type of injury, the gluteal and sciatic nerves may both be compromised at the sciatic notch. With sacral plexus lesions, the gluteal nerves, pudendal nerve, and posterior cutaneous nerve to the thigh may be affected. Once again, however, a sciatic notch injury may simultaneously involve all of these nerves where they exit the pelvis. The pudendal nerve is the furthest away from the sciatic nerve in the buttock; therefore, a deficit in this nerve may be the strongest evidence on examination of a sacral lesion. For sacral plexus injury patients, imaging and electrophysiological studies are usually required.

One common cause of a buttock-level sciatic lesion is an injection injury. The safest way to administer a buttock injection is to have the patient lie prone, and then place the injection in the upper outer quadrant. Standing bent over a sink or table, or rolling over in bed is not acceptable because the topographical anatomy of the buttock becomes distorted, especially in the elderly, who have reduced amounts of subcutaneous adipose tissue and sagging buttocks. The most dangerous injection quadrant is the superomedial one. Injections injuries are readily diagnosed, considering sciatic pain and deficits characteristically begin immediately after the offending injection. Occasionally, injection injuries can present minutes to hours after an injection; the cause of this delay is uncertain. Some believe it is irritation of the nerve by the offending substance being injected in or near the epineurium. Sciatic nerve injection injuries can cause severe motor and sensory deficits, or more commonly, a mild neurological deficit with persistent sciatica.

Other causes of buttock-level sciatic lesions include hip fractures and orthopedic procedures. This is because the sciatic nerve runs just dorsal to the hip joint, and is only separated from it by a few thin muscles. It is vulnerable to hematomas, adjacent hardware, intraoperative retraction or coagulation, and fracture/dislocations. Of note, when isolated hip fractures injure a peripheral nerve they usually only affect the sciatic nerve. In contrast, pelvic and sacral fractures often involve the sacral plexus. Penetrating trauma can also damage the sciatic nerve in the buttock region, but this is uncommon because the nerve is deep below the gluteus maximus.

Piriformis Syndrome

As described previously, upon exiting the pelvis, the sciatic nerve passes under the pyriformis muscle, which runs from the inner lateral margin of the sacrum to the greater trochanter of the femur (**Fig. 6–1**). Occasionally, the sciatic nerve runs over, or through, the pyriformis muscle. Definitive confirmation that pyriformis syndrome is a true clinical entity is pending, with many experts doubting its occurrence. Others have suggested pyriformis syndrome be categorized as neurogenic (with objective clinical findings) or non-neurogenic (without objective clinical findings). Patients with pyriformis syndrome have buttock and sciatic nerve distribution pain, usually without objective weakness or sensory loss on examination. Electrodiagnostic testing is usually normal. Many of these patients are originally thought to have lumbar disc herniations; either a normal lumbar spine magnetic resonance image (MRI) scan or failed spine surgery leads to the diagnosis of pyriformis syndrome. A steroid injection into the pyriformis muscle may help ascertain the diagnosis, but is not without risk. Pyriformis syndrome patients can have a history of a short fall and landing on their buttocks. If the patient is a woman and her symptoms are cyclical, one should consider focal nerve compression near the sciatic notch from endometriosis.

The Thigh

Complete and Partial Lesions

Injuries to the sciatic nerve in the thigh region are usually caused by gun shot wounds, and less commonly by lacerations. Femur fractures and/or repairs may also damage the sciatic nerve. Because the main branches to the hamstrings originate in the buttock region, even complete thigh-level sciatic lesions spare leg flexion. Although the tibial and peroneal divisions of the sciatic nerve do not split from one another until the lower third of the thigh, even upper thigh and buttock lesions may predominantly, or solely, involve just one of these divisions. This is because the tibial and peroneal divisions remain separate, even though they share a common epineurium as the sciatic nerve.

Compared with the tibial division, the peroneal division is more susceptible to injury. It is more commonly injured; the degree of injury is characteristically more severe; and recovery is less likely to occur. There are at least six potential reasons for this: (1) the peroneal division lies lateral and more superficial in the buttock region, making it more susceptible to trauma, (2) it is fixed between two anatomical points, the sciatic notch and lateral fibular head, unlike the tibial nerve, which is only fixed at the sciatic notch, (3) it has less blood supply than the tibial division, (4) it has fewer and larger fascicles with less intervening connective tissue (less tensile strength), (5) peroneal-innervated muscles (e.g., peroneus longus and brevis) are themselves concurrently injured with leg trauma, and (6) the peroneal division innervates long, thin extensor muscles, which often require robust reinnervation prior to them functioning.

The Knee/Leg

Tibial Palsy

A tibial palsy manifests as plantar flexion (gastrocnemius, soleus), foot inversion (tibialis posterior), toes flexion (flexor digitorum and hallucis longus, flexor digitorum and hallucis brevis), and foot intrinsic muscle weakness. Sensory loss occurs in the sole of the foot and the medial heel. Depending on the tibial division's contribution to the sural nerve, its sensory territory may also be affected. The most common causes of knee/leg tibial nerve injury are lacerations (knee level mostly) and tibial/ankle fracture or dislocations. Branches to the gastrocnemius and soleus muscles originate proximal to the tibial nerve's passage below these muscles. Therefore, when these muscles are weak, the lesion is in, or proximal to, the popliteal fossa. Sparing of the tibialis posterior (foot inversion) helps localize a tibial lesion to the deep posterior compartment of the mid-leg or below. Furthermore, sparing of the flexors digitorum and hallucis longus places the lesion to the lower third of the leg or distal to the tarsal tunnel. Baker's cysts or other mass lesions can also cause tibial palsies at the knee. Without a history of trauma, the examiner should thoroughly palpate the popliteal fossa for masses.

Common Peroneal Nerve Palsy

The usual type of peroneal nerve damage at the knee/leg is a stretch/contusion injury, usually with a concomitant fracture (usually sports related). Damage to this nerve is not uncommon because it is superficial and in a fixed position at the lateral fibular head. Of note, peroneal nerve palsy is the most common lower-extremity nerve injury occurring after trauma. Tribiofibular joint ganglion cysts, adjacent or even within the common peroneal nerve, may also cause a peroneal division deficit at the knee.

Idiopathic entrapment of the common peroneal nerve occurs below the fibrous edge of the peroneus longus muscle at the fibular head, the *fibular tunnel* (**Fig. 6–25**). Diabetics are especially prone to this problem. When this occurs, both the superficial and deep peroneal branches are involved to a variable degree. Sometimes, an isolated palsy to the deep peroneal nerve may occur when this branch passes under the fibrous edge of the extensor digitorum longus muscle. Common peroneal nerve entrapment patients have pain and numbness in a peroneal distribution (i.e., over the dorsum of the foot), radiating down from the fibular head. The lateral cutaneous nerve of the calf is spared because it does not pass through the fibular tunnel. Weakness of foot dorsiflexion (tibialis anterior), foot eversion (peroneus longus and brevis), and toe extension (extensor digitorum longus, extensor hallucis longus, and extensor digitorum brevis) may occur with more severe lesions. A Tinel's sign is often present at the fibular head. Peroneal entrapment at the fibular head must be carefully differentiated from a L5 radiculopathy. In this situation, an electrodiagnostic consult is especially useful because the tibialis posterior is predominantly innervated by the L5 spinal nerve via the tibial nerve, not the common peroneal nerve.

Strawberry picker's palsy occurs in persons who spend extended periods in the squatting position, which causes bilateral common peroneal nerve compression at the fibular heads. External trauma affecting the common peroneal nerve at the

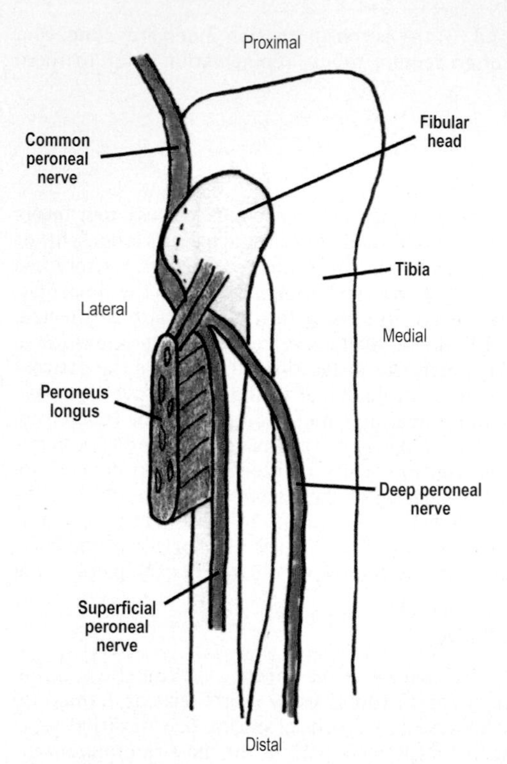

Figure 6–25 Peroneal nerve entrapment at the fibular head. Idiopathic entrapment of the common peroneal nerve may occur at the fibular head when this nerve passes below the fibrous edge of the peroneus longus muscle. Sometimes, an isolated palsy involving the deep peroneal nerve may occur when this branch passes under the fibrous edge of the extensor digitorum longus muscle.

fibular head may occur more frequently in persons who quickly lose weight (*slimmer's paralysis*). This is thought to be because with weight loss the adipose tissue that usually pads the common peroneal nerve is reduced, and furthermore, the patient now is able to cross his or her legs, something that was more difficult when the patient was heavier. Postpartum foot drop is also a known phenomenon, having a variety of causes. These include L5 radiculopathy, pressure upon the lumbosacral trunk where it passes over the bony margin of the sacroiliac joint, external compression of the common peroneal nerve or its branches by the leg holders in the lithotomy position, and in certain developing countries, from prolonged squatting.

- **Posttraumatic compartment syndrome in the leg may involve the anterior, posterior, and/or peroneal (lateral) compartments, producing isolated nerve palsies in the deep peroneal, tibial, and superficial peroneal branches, respectively.**

The Foot

Foot Drop

Isolated foot drop, or more specifically weakness in the tibialis anterior, extensor hallucis longus, and peroneus muscles, is caused by nerve injury in a variety of locations, including the L5 spinal nerve, lumbosacral trunk, peroneal (lateral) division of the sciatic nerve in the buttock or thigh, and the common peroneal nerve. Although an adequate history may be the most useful way to make the diagnosis, the clinical examination supplemented with electromyography can be confirmatory. For example, both L5 radicular and lumbosacral trunk lesions should cause tibialis posterior and gluteal muscle weakness. However, compared with L5 radicular lesions, patients with lumbosacral trunk damage usually do not have paraspinal muscle denervation on electromyography. Patients with peroneal division sciatic injury should have denervation of the short head of the biceps femoris, with all the other hamstrings being normal. It is rarely possible to observe short head weakness during muscular testing when the long head of the biceps femoris is functioning. In this situation, electromyography is useful.

Tarsal Tunnel Syndrome

Tarsal tunnel syndrome is an uncommon entrapment involving the medial and lateral plantar nerves where they run under the flexor retinaculum, which is a ligament that connects the medial malleolus to the calcaneus (**Fig. 6–3**). Patients with this syndrome commonly have a history of regional ankle trauma, and therefore postinjury fibrosis may be a common cause. Other etiologies include systemic disorders (e.g., rheumatoid arthritis and diabetes mellitus). Patients with tarsal tunnel syndrome complain of sole pain, numbness, and/or paresthesias, which are worsened with walking and standing but relieved with rest and elevation. The pain usually is localized to the metatarsals. Heel pain is uncommon. Pinprick, vibratory sense, and two-point discrimination can be abnormal. Complaints of weakness are uncommon, but when present, involve the foot intrinsics. A Tinel's sign may be present posterior to the medial malleolus, possibly radiating down into the foot. Percussion may also cause pain radiating *up* the course of the tibial nerve, known as the *Valleix phenomenon*. Peripheral neuropathy may be differentiated from tarsal tunnel syndrome because the former usually has sensory loss outside the territory of the tibial nerve (e.g., in the sural or saphenous nerves), as well as absent ankle jerks (the foot flexors are innervated proximal to the tarsal tunnel). Nerve conduction studies are used to help confirm the diagnosis of tarsal tunnel syndrome.

Anterior tarsal tunnel syndrome is a very rare cause of distal deep peroneal nerve entrapment under one, or both, extensor retinaculums on the dorsum of the foot (**Fig. 6–26**). Patients have extensor digitorum brevis muscle mass weakness (and/or wasting) on examination, report a dull ache on the dorsum of the foot, and sometimes have numbness localized to their first web space. A Tinel's sign may occur. Tight-fitting shoes or local fibrosis following trauma may be causative.

Morton's Neuroma

Morton's neuroma is actually not a neuroma, but the chronic irritation of a common plantar nerve, usually the one innervating the third web space. This nerve is usually made up of branches from both the medial and lateral plantar nerves, and is pinched repetitively between the third and fourth metatarsal heads where this nerve runs under the deep transverse metatarsal ligament (**Fig. 6–27**). Focal swelling of the nerve occurs secondary to intraneural fibrosis.

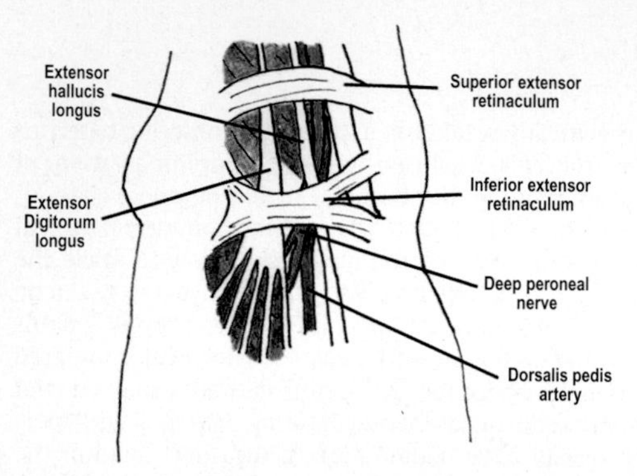

Figure 6–26 Anterior tarsal tunnel anatomy (dorsal view). This syndrome is a very rare cause of distal, deep peroneal nerve entrapment under one, or both, extensor retinaculums on the dorsum of the foot. Patients have dorsal foot discomfort, numbness in the first web space, and possible wasting of the extensor digitorum brevis.

Patients with a Morton's neuroma have pain between the third and fourth metatarsals, which radiates to the third and fourth toes. The pain is worsened with walking, relieved by rest and elevation, and usually does not occur at night. Squeezing the metatarsals together can cause a shooting pain into the third and fourth toes. A Tinel's sign may be present. An ultrasound examination can help make the diagnosis.

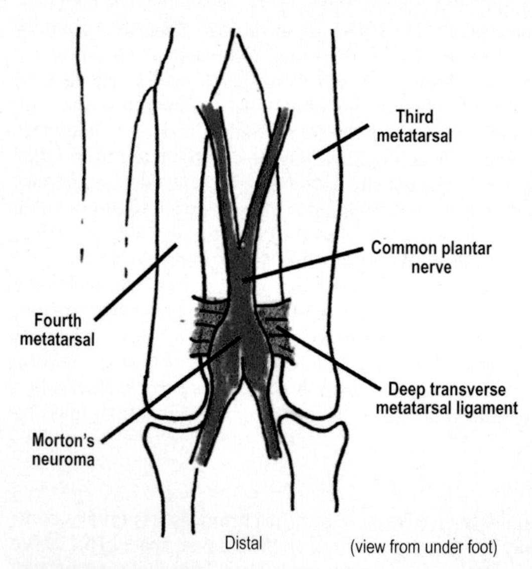

Figure 6–27 Morton's neuroma. This is actually the chronic irritation of a common plantar nerve, usually the one innervating the third web space, which causes perineural fibrosis, *not* aneuroma. The affected nerve is pinched repetitively where it runs between the third and fourth metatarsals under the deep transverse metatarsal ligament.

7

The Diagnostic Anatomy of the Inguinal Complex of Nerves

Originating in the lumbar plexus (T12 to L4), several peripheral nerves course distally through the inguinal region to provide motor and sensory innervation to the groin and thigh. Although damage of these nerves is uncommon, certain types of idiopathic, iatrogenic, and traumatic injuries may occur. Therefore, their anatomy and possible deficits remain important and will be discussed in this chapter.

The two major nerves of the inguinal complex are the femoral and obturator nerves, which are the primary output of the lumbar plexus. The lateral femoral cutaneous nerve, irritation of which causes meralgia paresthetica, as well as other nerves in the inguinal and genital region, will also be described. The inguinal complex of nerves controls thigh flexion, thigh adduction, and leg extension. Sensory coverage includes the groin, anterior and medial thigh, and the medial leg down to the arch of the foot.

♦ Anatomical Course

A general overview of the inguinal complex of nerves' anatomical relationships with the iliopsoas muscles, pelvis, and inguinal ligament is illustrated in **Fig. 7–1**.

The Femoral Nerve

The femoral nerve is the largest branch of the lumbar plexus, being composed of the posterior divisions of the L2, L3, and L4 ventral rami. The anterior divisions of these ventral rami make up the obturator nerve (see below). These divisional contributions to the femoral nerve merge posterior to the *psoas major* muscle, and anterior to the transverse processes of the spine. Once formed, the femoral nerve runs inferiorly and laterally, in an oblique course down the pelvis, remaining under but near the lateral margin of the psoas major. The femoral nerve emerges from under the psoas major at the groove this muscle forms with the iliacus in the pelvis, approximately 4 cm proximal to the inguinal ligament. When the femoral nerve exits from under the psoas and passes over the iliacus muscle, it remains below the rigid iliacus fascia, which forms the roof of the *iliacus compartment*.

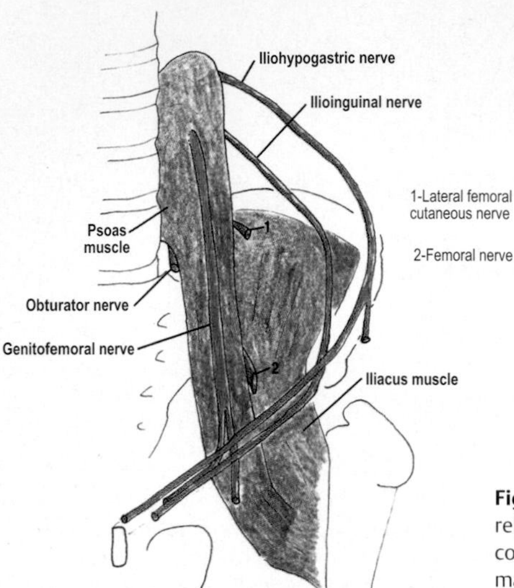

Figure 7–1 General anatomical relationships between the inguinal complex of nerves and the psoas major, iliacus, pelvic rim, abdominal wall, and inguinal ligament.

The femoral nerve passes deep to the inguinal ligament to enter the femoral triangle of the anterior thigh, where it remains lateral to the femoral artery (**Fig. 7–2**). The femoral triangle is bordered by the inguinal ligament superiorly, the sartorius muscle laterally and inferiorly, and the adductor longus muscle medially. The femoral nerve lies deep to the iliacus fascia, which extends from the pelvis to cover and protect the femoral triangle. Of note, a small window in the iliacus fascia is present over the femoral vein and medial half of the femoral artery, just below the inguinal ligament.

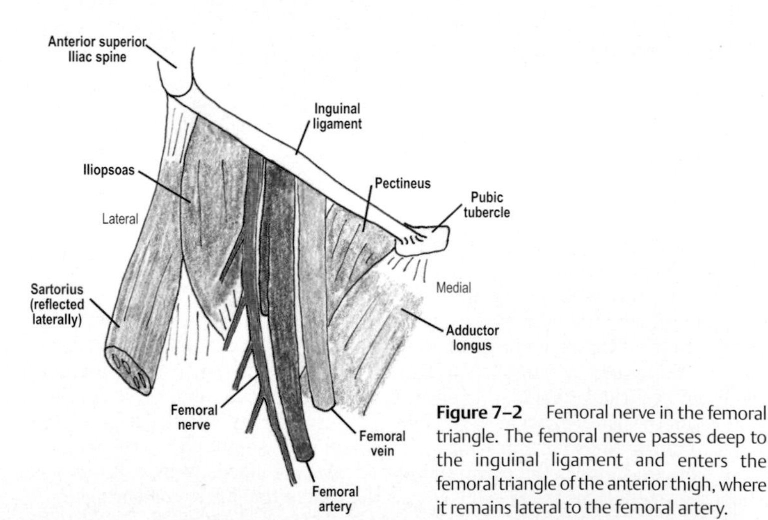

Figure 7–2 Femoral nerve in the femoral triangle. The femoral nerve passes deep to the inguinal ligament and enters the femoral triangle of the anterior thigh, where it remains lateral to the femoral artery.

A few centimeters distal to the inguinal ligament, under the sartorius muscle, the femoral nerve almost immediately splits into numerous terminal branches. These branches include three cutaneous sensory branches: the medial femoral cutaneous, the intermediate femoral cutaneous, and the saphenous nerve. The remaining branches are motor nerves to the quadriceps, sartorius, and pectineus. The quadriceps is composed of four muscles: the rectus femoris, vastus lateralis, vastus intermedialis, and vastus medialis. A common branch to the rectus femoris and vastus lateralis usually originates very proximal, and runs with the lateral femoral circumflex artery.

The saphenous nerve continues distally in a gradual, oblique course, from the femoral nerve near the inguinal ligament toward the medial knee. The saphenous nerve runs with the femoral artery and vein, deep and parallel to the sartorius muscle, along a groove between the adductor longus and vastus medialis (subsartorial canal). The saphenous nerve then enters the adductor canal (of Hunter) with the femoral vessels, but instead of passing into the posterior compartment of the leg, the saphenous nerve remains anteromedial to the knee. The saphenous nerve pierces the subcutaneous fascia at, or just distal to, the knee. It provides sensory coverage to the medial leg, medial malleolus, and arch of the foot.

The Obturator Nerve

The obturator nerve is the second major nerve from the lumbar plexus, arising from the anterior divisions of the L2, L3, and L4 ventral rami. These spinal nerve contributions fuse to form the obturator nerve in the substance of the psoas major. Once formed, the obturator nerve makes it way under the psoas major to this muscle's inferomedial border, and from there runs between the psoas and the iliac vessels through the pelvis toward the obturator foramen (**Fig. 7–1**). The large obturator foramen is mostly covered by the obturator membrane, upon which the obturator externus muscle originates. A hole in the obturator membrane near the most superolateral aspect of the foramen is called the *obturator canal*. The obturator nerve exits the pelvis via the obturator canal (**Fig. 7–3**).

Just prior to exiting the pelvis, the obturator nerve bifurcates into an anterior (superficial) and posterior division. Both of these obturator divisions pass through the obturator canal and perforate the obturator externus muscle, which runs from the obturator membrane to the proximal femur. Once piercing this muscle, these two divisions run deep to the pectineus muscle. The smaller, and deeper, posterior division branches upon the obturator externus, sending some branches under the adductor brevis to innervate a portion of the adductor magnus, a muscle that is also innervated by the tibial division of the sciatic nerve. The more superficial, anterior division runs over the adductor brevis upon which it ramifies. The anterior division passes deep to the adductor longus.

A cutaneous sensory branch from the anterior division originates quite proximally, usually where this division ramifies on the adductor brevis. This cutaneous branch passes deep to the adductor longus with an oblique trajectory toward the medial, inner thigh.

- **In a third of the population, an *accessory obturator nerve* is present, which originates from the anterior divisions of the L3 and L4 ventral rami. These patients have a normal, albeit smaller than usual, obturator nerve that follows its standard anatomical course. The accessory obturator nerve forms in the substance of the psoas major and passes with the normal obturator nerve medial to the psoas toward the obturator foramen.**

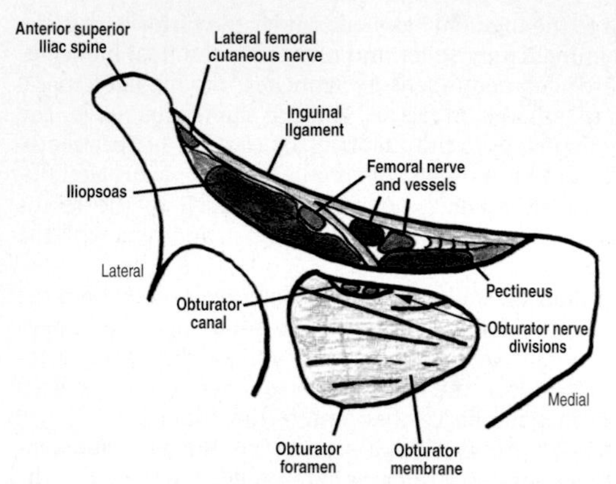

Figure 7–3 Cross-sectional view of the inguinal region from an anterior/inferior perspective. Structures that run from the pelvis to the thigh under the inguinal ligament are depicted. The obturator nerve's divisions are shown passing through the obturator canal, which is formed by the obturator membrane and is located in the superolateral portion of the larger, bony obturator foramen.

However, the accessory obturator nerve does not pass through the obturator canal, but instead passes over the superior pubic ramus. Once over the ramus, this nerve dives below the pectineus muscle to anastomose with the anterior division of the obturator nerve. When present, the accessory obturator nerve innervates the pectineus muscle, which usually receives its innervation from the femoral nerve.

The Lateral Femoral Cutaneous Nerve

The lateral femoral cutaneous nerve originates from the posterior divisions of the L2 and L3 ventral rami, just prior to where these two elements join the posterior division of L4 to form the femoral nerve. The lateral femoral cutaneous nerve travels out from under the psoas major, looping around and upon the superior portion of the iliacus muscle toward the anterosuperior iliac crest. This nerve then exits the pelvis just medial to the anterosuperior iliac crest, underneath the most lateral portion of the inguinal ligament. The lateral femoral cutaneous nerve usually passes under the inguinal ligament approximately 2 cm medial to the anterosuperior iliac spine.

Once outside the pelvis, this nerve immediately splits into two or more branches, pierces the fascia, and then runs subcutaneous over the lateral aspect of the thigh. The lateral femoral cutaneous nerve and its branches usually run superficial to the sartorius muscle.

- **The course of the lateral femoral cutaneous nerve in the region of the anterosuperior iliac spine is variable. The nerve can pass over the iliac crest, over the inguinal ligament, or even through a small hiatus in the ligament itself (Fig. 7–4). These variations are thought to predispose an individual to idiopathic entrapment of this nerve near the iliac crest (meralgia paresthetica). The lateral femoral cutaneous nerve may also run under or through the sartorius muscle. It may even originate, in part, from the femoral or genitofemoral nerves.**

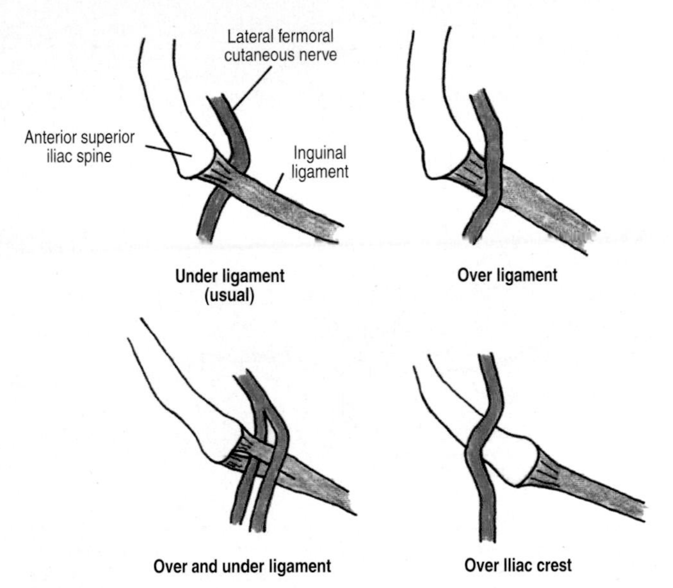

Figure 7–4 Lateral femoral cutaneous nerve at the anterosuperior iliac spine. The lateral femoral cutaneous nerve usually exits the pelvis just medial to the anterosuperior iliac crest, underneath the most lateral portion of the inguinal ligament. In this region, variations in its course are the rule, with the more common ones illustrated.

Other Nerves of the Inguinal Region

The ventral rami of T12 and L1 form a common trunk under the psoas major. This trunk then splits into the *iliohypogastric* and *ilioinguinal nerves*, with the iliohypogastric being the more superior of the two. These nerves run mostly parallel to each other, first passing through the psoas major, and then piercing its lateral margin to run over the quadratus lumborum muscle.

The iliohypogastric nerve perforates the transversus abdominis muscle over the iliac crest, and runs around the flank between this muscle and the internal oblique. Immediately superior to the anterosuperior iliac spine, a lateral branch of the iliohypogastric nerve perforates both the internal and external oblique muscles to become subcutaneous to innervate the superior lateral gluteal region. The remaining portion of the iliohypogastric nerve continues toward the midline, entering the distal inguinal canal, and passing through the superficial inguinal ring to become subcutaneous in the hypogastric/suprapubic region (**Fig. 7–5**).

The ilioinguinal nerve also passes around the flank toward the inguinal region, just caudal to the iliohypogastric nerve. The ilioinguinal nerve, however, pierces *both* the transversus abdominis and internal oblique muscles to run between the latter and the external oblique. This nerve gives sensory branches as it runs adjacent to the spermatic cord and cremaster muscle in the inguinal canal, eventually becoming subcutaneous with the medial branch of the iliohypogastric nerve through the superficial inguinal ring (**Fig. 7–5**).

The *genitofemoral nerve* is made up of branches from the L1 and L2 spinal nerves. Once formed, this nerve passes through the psoas major muscle and perforates its anterior margin just medial to the psoas minor muscle (when present). The genitofemoral

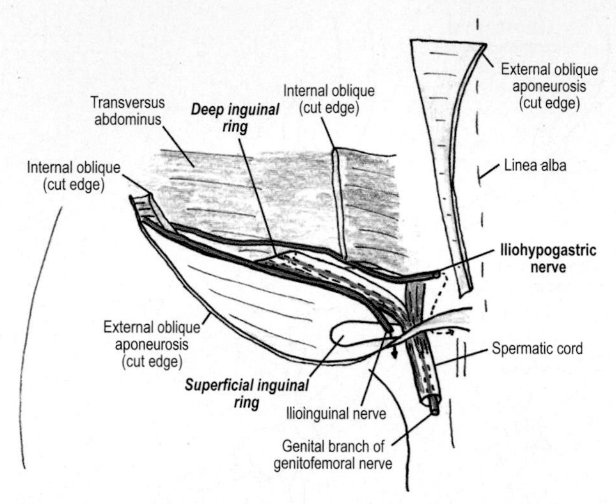

Figure 7–5 Course of the iliohypogastric, ilioinguinal, and genitofemoral nerves in the inguinal canal (right side, anterior view). The genitofemoral nerve runs along the psoas muscle and splits into a femoral and genital branch. The femoral branch passes under the inguinal ligament, while the genital branch enters the deep inguinal ring to pass distally within the spermatic cord. Portions of both the iliohypogastric and ilioinguinal nerves also pass within the inguinal canal, but not within the spermatic cord.

nerve then passes distally adjacent to the ureter, eventually splitting into a genital and femoral branch just proximal to the inguinal ligament. The femoral branch passes under the inguinal ligament just lateral to the femoral artery, becoming subcutaneous in the femoral triangle (**Fig. 7–5**). The genital branch enters the deep inguinal ring, passes through the inguinal canal within the spermatic cord, and emerges from the superficial inguinal ring to innervate a portion of the genitalia.

♦ **A common variation is for the ilioinguinal and iliohypogastric nerves to be derived only from the L1 spinal nerve, not T12.**

♦ Motor Innervation and Testing

The Femoral Nerve

The femoral nerve controls thigh flexion at the hip, and leg extension at the knee (**Fig. 7–6**). The first muscle innervated by the femoral nerve is the *psoas major*. Co-innervation to this muscle also arises directly from the lumbar plexus (ventral rami). The second muscle innervated by the femoral nerve is the *iliacus*, which is in the pelvis. These two muscles, along with the psoas minor, when present, insert into the proximal femur to mediate thigh flexion at the hip. These muscles, collectively termed the *iliopsoas* (L2-L4), are tested together by having the patient raise the thigh against resistance (**Fig. 7–7**). The patient should be either seated or supine.

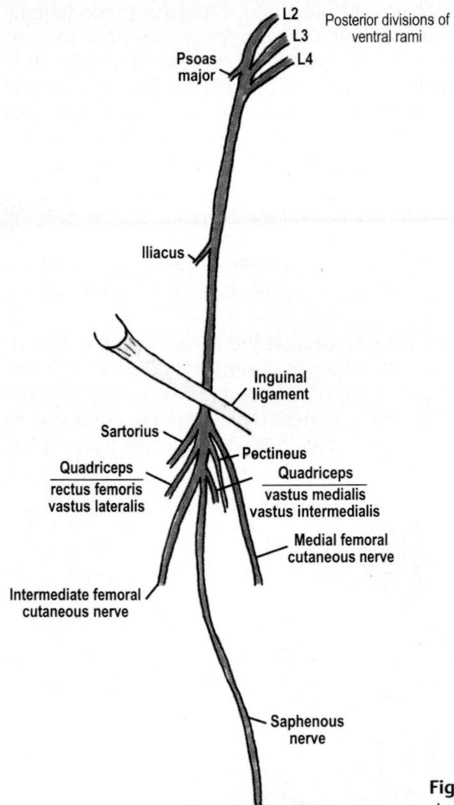

Figure 7–6 Motor innervation from the femoral nerve (L2–L4).

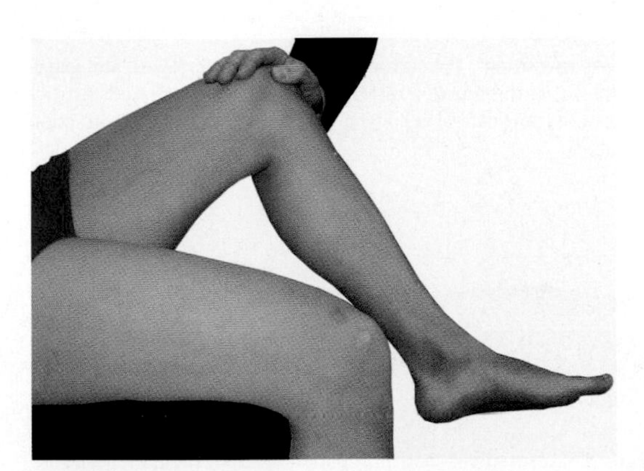

Figure 7–7 Iliopsoas (L2-L4) assessment: The psoas major and iliacus muscles (collectively termed the iliopsoas) are tested together by having the patient raise the knee (flex the thigh) against resistance, with the patient either sitting (shown) or lying supine.

Upon entering the femoral triangle and branching extensively, the femoral nerve innervates the *pectineus*, *sartorius*, and *quadriceps* muscles (L2-L4). The pectineus runs from the anterior pelvic rim (near the pubic tubercle) to the proximal femur. Together, the pectineus, psoas major, and iliacus, form the floor of the femoral triangle, with the latter two muscles lying deeper and more lateral than the pectineus. The pectineus cannot be isolated on exam, and therefore is not discussed further. The sartorius, or tailor's muscle, runs from the anterosuperior iliac spine, obliquely down the leg to the medial knee, inserting into the anterior tibial tubercle. The sartorius muscle has a complex function, but in essence, abducts, flexes, and externally rotates the thigh. To semi-isolate this muscle, start by having the patient seated. Then instruct him or her to place the foot on the contralateral knee by dragging it up the shin (**Fig. 7–8**). Contraction of the sartorius may be palpated.

The quadriceps muscles mediate leg extension at the knee. The *rectus femoris* and *vastus lateralis* often share a common branch of the femoral nerve; the *vastus intermedialis* and *medialis* usually have their own branches (they also can share a common branch). With the patient seated, the quadriceps are tested by applying resistance against leg extension (**Fig. 7–9**). The muscle mass of the

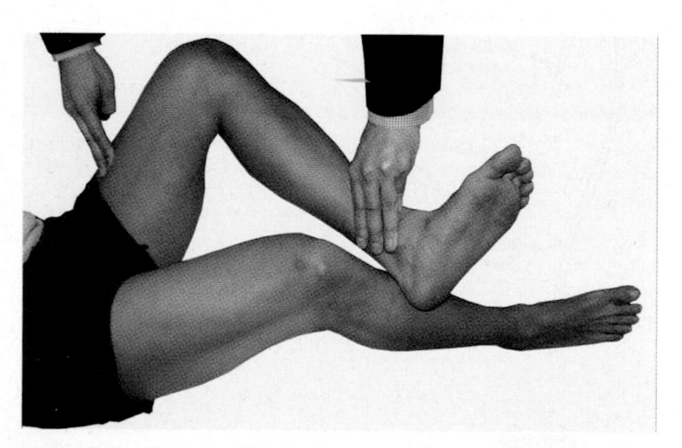

Figure 7–8 Sartorius (L2-L4) assessment: The sartorius muscle abducts, flexes, and externally rotates the thigh. To semi-isolate this muscle, start by having the patient seated. Instruct him or her to place the foot on the contralateral knee by dragging it up the shin. Contraction of the sartorius may be palpated.

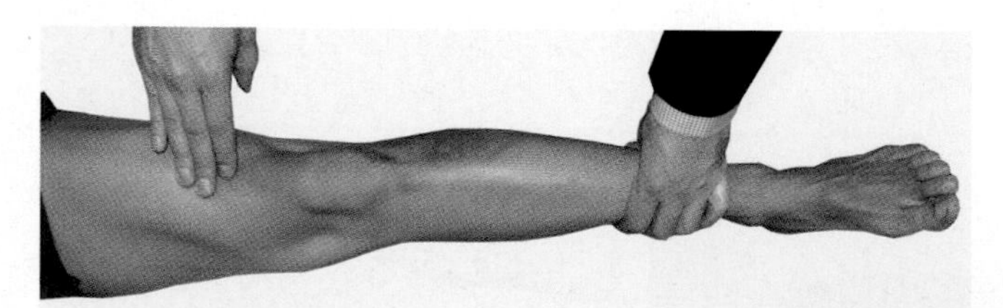

Figure 7–9 Quadriceps (L2-L4) assessment: With the patient seated, the quadriceps are tested by applying resistance against leg extension. The quadriceps' muscle mass should be observed and palpated because the sartorius (femoral nerve) and tensor fascia lata (superior gluteal nerve) may substitute for leg extension.

quadriceps should be observed and palpated because the sartorius (femoral nerve) and tensor fascia lata (superior gluteal nerve) may deceptively substitute for leg extension in some patients.

The Obturator Nerve

The anterior division of the obturator nerve provides motor fibers to the *adductor brevis*, *adductor longus*, and *gracilis* (**Fig. 7–10**). This pattern of muscular innervation makes sense, considering the obturator's anterior division runs between the first two muscles and ends near the third. The posterior division innervates the *obturator externus*, and terminates by innervating a small portion of the *adductor magnus*, deep to the adductor brevis. To test obturator nerve motor function (i.e., the adductors, L2-L4), have the patient squeeze the thighs together with resistance placed at the inner knees (**Fig. 7–11**).

♦ **Innervation of the adductors is variable, with the adductors longus, brevis, and magnus often receiving innervation from both, or either, divisions of the obturator nerve.**

Other Nerves of the Inguinal Region

The iliohypogastric and ilioinguinal nerves provide motor branches to the transversus abdominis and internal oblique muscles. The ilioinguinal nerve also innervates the pyramidalis muscle, which, when present, can be tested with electromyography. The genital branch of the genitofemoral nerve innervates the cremaster muscle, which helps mediate testicular thermoregulation by elevating the ipsilateral testicle. This reflex may be tested by applying light touch to the

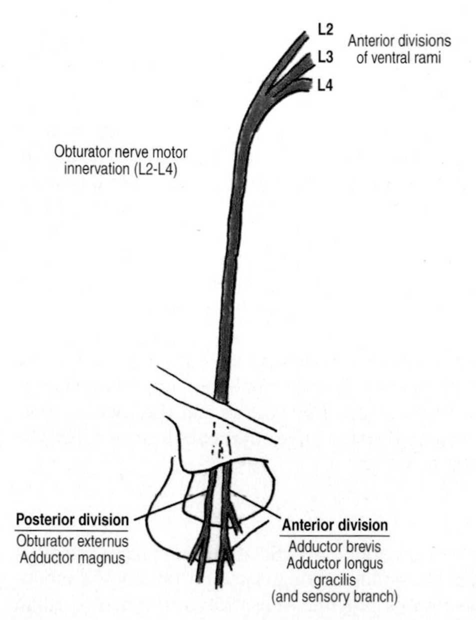

Figure 7–10 Motor innervation from the obturator nerve.

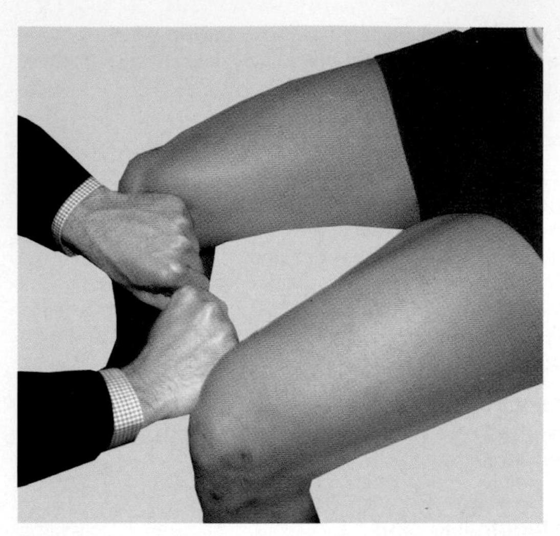

Figure 7–11 Adductor (L2-L4) assessment: Have the patient squeeze the thighs with resistance placed at the inner knees.

inguinal region and observing ipsilateral testicular elevation. The cremaster reflex is an unreliable clinical finding, however.

♦ Sensory Innervation

The Femoral Nerve

The femoral nerve's sensory territory includes the anterior and medial thigh, as well as the medial leg and foot via the saphenous nerve (**Fig. 7–12**). The *medial femoral cutaneous nerve* branches from the femoral nerve in the femoral triangle and carries sensation from the medial thigh, mostly from the distal medial thigh (the proximal, medial thigh is covered more by the obturator nerve). The *intermediate femoral cutaneous nerve* also branches from the proximal femoral nerve in the thigh and covers sensation on the anterior (and somewhat medial) aspect of the thigh. Overall, an autonomous sensory zone for the femoral nerve is over the distal, anterior thigh.

The *saphenous nerve's* sensory territory includes the medial knee, medial leg, medial malleolus, and the arch of the foot. Mostly small, unnamed branches of the saphenous nerve provide this cutaneous innervation. On the medial knee, however, the saphenous nerve frequently has a large cutaneous branch called the *infrapatellar branch of the saphenous nerve.*

The Obturator Nerve

As mentioned, the obturator nerve's anterior (superficial) division has a proximal sensory branch that passes under the adductor longus and perforates the subcutaneous fascia of the thigh. This branch provides sensation to the medial thigh region (**Fig. 7–13**). Sensory loss in this area is not always present with complete obturator palsies, and therefore is not considered autonomous.

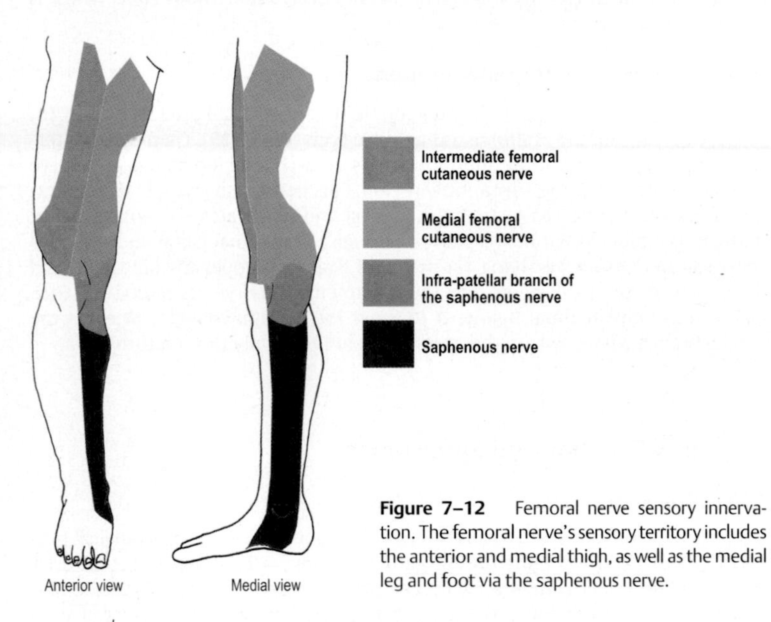

Figure 7–12 Femoral nerve sensory innervation. The femoral nerve's sensory territory includes the anterior and medial thigh, as well as the medial leg and foot via the saphenous nerve.

Figure 7–13 Obturator nerve sensory innervation (medial view). The obturator nerve's anterior (superficial) division has a proximal sensory branch that passes under the adductor longus and perforates the fascia of the thigh. This branch provides sensation to the medial thigh region.

The Lateral Femoral Cutaneous Nerve

The lateral femoral cutaneous nerve's sensory territory includes the anterior, lateral aspect of the thigh (**Fig. 7–14**). This nerve has an autonomous zone, which is located on the mid-lateral thigh.

Other Nerves of the Inguinal Region

The iliohypogastric, ilioinguinal, and genitofemoral nerves all provide significant sensory coverage of the inguinal and pubic regions (**Fig. 7–15**). Their sensory territories overlap, but semi-autonomous zones do exist. The iliohypogastric nerve provides sensation to the suprapubic region. This nerve also gives a lateral cutaneous branch that passes over the iliac crest and innervates the upper, lateral buttock. The ilioinguinal nerve passes through the inguinal canal and provides sensation to the skin overlying the inguinal ligament, upper medial thigh, and mons pubis/base of the penis. For the genitofemoral nerve, its femoral branch passes under the inguinal ligament to cover the femoral triangle, whereas the genital branch passes within the spermatic cord to supply the scrotum/labia.

♦ Clinical Findings and Syndromes

The Femoral Nerve

Injury to the femoral nerve is usually iatrogenic. Causes include gynecological procedures, femoral artery puncture for catheterization, arterial bypass procedures, hip surgery using methylmethacrylate, and pelvic surgery for tumors. Traditionally, an abdominal hysterectomy is the operation most frequently associated with

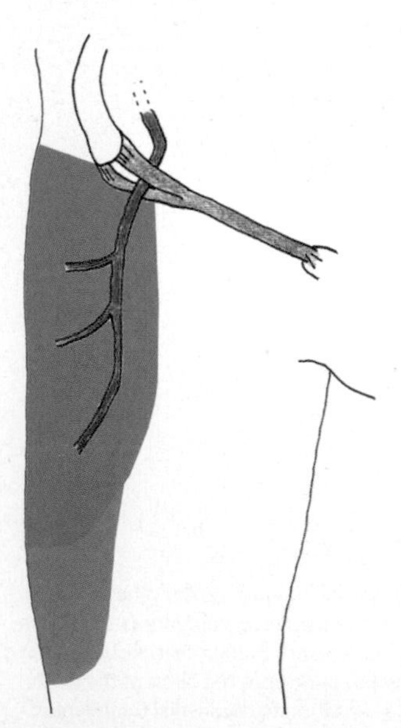

Figure 7–14 Lateral femoral cutaneous nerve sensory innervation. This nerve's sensory territory includes the anterolateral aspect of the thigh. This nerve has an autonomous zone, which is located on the lower, lateral thigh proximal to the knee.

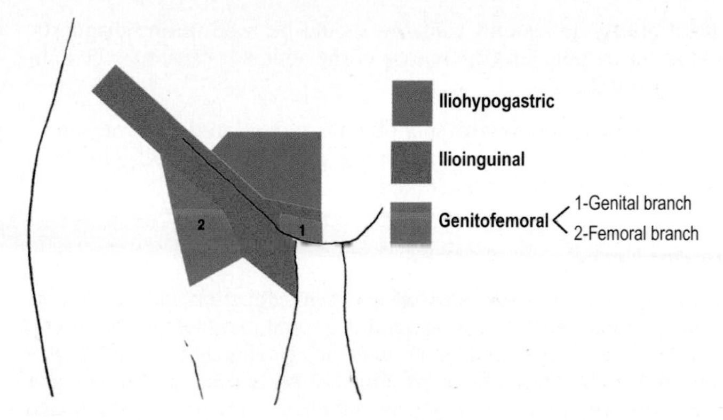

Figure 7–15 Sensory territory of the iliohypogastric, ilioinguinal, and genitofemoral nerves. These nerves all provide significant sensory coverage of the inguinal and pubic regions. Although their coverage overlaps, semi-autonomous zones do exist. For the iliohypogastric nerve, it is the suprapubic region. For the ilioinguinal nerve, it is the inguinal ligament region. For the genitofemoral nerve, it is the femoral triangle (femoral branch) and scrotum/labia (genital branch).

femoral nerve damage. Trauma may also cause femoral nerve injury, including gunshot wounds to the groin and pelvis, lacerations, and hip/pelvis fractures. Expanding retroperitoneal (psoas or iliacus compartment) and femoral triangle hematomas from anticoagulation, trauma, or catheter placement may also cause femoral injury. Although proximal diabetic neuropathies frequently involve the femoral nerve, this nerve is rarely affected in isolation. Usually the lumbar spinal nerves, the lumbosacral plexus, and other peripheral nerves are involved simultaneously.

Patients with significant femoral neuropathies often complain of incoordination or buckling of the knee and not paralysis per se. These patients have the most trouble standing from a seated position, as well as climbing stairs. A frontward kick is not possible. Sensory loss may be confirmatory, and includes the anterior thigh (intermediate femoral cutaneous nerve), lower medial thigh (medial femoral cutaneous nerve), medial knee (infrapatellar branch of the saphenous nerve), and medial leg and foot (saphenous nerve).

For patients with a suspected femoral neuropathy involving the iliopsoas muscle, which indicates a very proximal lesion, one should make certain to examine thigh adductor strength. If thigh adduction is weak, a lesion affecting the lumbar plexus, or multiple spinal nerves (i.e., L2–L4), is more likely. Imaging should be performed. Furthermore, a femoral neuropathy should be differentiated from a L4 radiculopathy. Both femoral neuropathy and L4 radiculopathy can manifest with quadriceps weakness, an absent knee jerk, and medial leg (shin) numbness in the saphenous territory. However, only a radiculopathy would have concurrent thigh adductor (L2–L4), anterior tibialis (L4–S1), and posterior tibialis (L4–L5) weakness. Therefore, these three muscles should also be closely examined in these patients.

Idiopathic entrapment of the saphenous nerve has been reported at the adductor canal in the distal, medial thigh. Prolonged or absent sensory conduction velocities in the saphenous nerve distal to the canal may occur. To avoid damage to the femoral artery, ultrasound guidance should be used during diagnostic nerve blocks in this region. Surgical release of the adductor canal may be indicated for select patients.

- **Rarely, patients may present with spontaneous and isolated numbness in the territory of the saphenous nerve's infrapatellar branch (i.e., *gonyalgia paresthetica*). The cause is uncertain.**

The Obturator Nerve

Patients with obturator palsies have weak thigh adduction and a variable amount of medial thigh sensory loss. The adductor tendon reflex may be absent, although this reflex may be absent in normal subjects. Injury to the obturator nerve is rare, but may be caused by penetrating trauma to the inguinal region or pelvis. As with the femoral nerve, iatrogenic etiologies are most common, and occur after pelvic surgery, especially for tumors. These injuries may be from direct manipulation or transection of the nerve, or more commonly, from a retractor stretch injury. Sometimes motor and sensory deficits are minimal to absent, and the patient only complains of pelvic/groin pain radiating to the medial thigh. If a neuroma occurs in this latter case, then a Tinel's sign may be present in the groin or lateral vaginal wall. Injury to the accessory obturator nerve may also occur where it passes over the superior pubic ramus.

To exclude a lumbar plexus lesion, or radiculopathy (e.g., L3, L4), in patients with suspected obturator palsies, normal strength in the quadriceps and an active knee jerk should be documented.

Idiopathic obturator nerve entrapment by a fibrous arch in the obturator canal has been reported. These patients present with groin discomfort and pain radiating to the medial thigh. Although adductor strength is often normal in these patients, needle electromyography of the thigh adductors may help confirm the diagnosis. A test infiltration of anesthetic where the nerve is most tender may be both therapeutically and diagnostically useful.

The Lateral Femoral Cutaneous Nerve (Barnhardt–Roth Syndrome)

Irritation of the lateral femoral cutaneous nerve is referred to as *meralgia paresthetica* (Barnhardt–Roth syndrome). Patients report numbness, paresthesias, pain, and/or hyperesthesia on the anterolateral aspect of the thigh. The etiology of this syndrome is usually considered idiopathic; however, it can often be related to repetitive, minor trauma or irritation. Patients sometimes report worse pain with standing and walking, and relief with flexion at the hip or sitting. Most symptoms are mild and self-limiting. Examination reveals sensory changes, especially hyperesthesia, on the lateral thigh. One provocative examination maneuver is to extend the thigh at the hip, which places the nerve on stretch and may thereby exacerbate the patient's symptoms. Deep palpation along the lateral inguinal ligament may be tender. A Tinel's sign is usually absent. The diagnosis may be confirmed with an injection of local anesthetic, which should ameliorate the symptoms. However, considering the anatomical variability this nerve exhibits (**Fig. 7–4**), there are many false-negatives with this test. Sensory conduction velocities may aid in the diagnosis.

An anomalous course of the lateral femoral cutaneous nerve may predispose one to neuropathy. Other predisposing conditions include obesity, ascites, and pregnancy: The protuberant abdomen is thought to distort regional anatomy and predispose one to meralgia paresthetica. Conversely, extreme weight loss is also associated with this disorder. Diabetes does not appear to be related. An autosomal dominant form of familial meralgia paresthetica has been reported.

An isolated neuropathy of the lateral femoral cutaneous nerve can be readily differentiated from a femoral or lumbar plexus lesion because the latter diagnoses cause more extensive sensory loss over the anterior/medial thigh, as well as motor weakness. The more problematic differential is that from a L2 radiculopathy, which affects the upper, lateral thigh. However, a L2 radiculopathy causes pain or numbness extending more over the anterior and medial aspect of the upper thigh than expected in meralgia paresthetica. Furthermore, a L2 radiculopathy may also cause iliopsoas weakness.

Inguinal Neuralgia

The iliohypogastric and ilioinguinal nerves may be disrupted or damaged secondary to transverse abdominal incisions (e.g., hysterectomies or other lower quadrant procedures), or during inguinal hernia repairs. Damage to either nerve may cause back, inguinal, and scrotal/labial pain. To confirm the diagnosis of an iliohypogastric or ilioinguinal neuropathy, three criteria should be fulfilled: (1) history of a surgical procedure involving the abdomen or pelvis, (2) sensory changes in the suprapubic (iliohypogastric nerve) or along the inguinal ligament (ilioinguinal nerve), and (3) anesthetic infiltration of these nerves near the anterosuperior iliac spine produces relief. As mentioned, sensory testing in the groin helps distinguish which of these two nerves is involved.

Although rare, the genitofemoral nerve may be damaged during inguinal hernia repair or gynecological procedures. Previous appendicitis or psoas abscesses can also damage this nerve on the anterior margin of the psoas muscle. Genitofemoral neuralgia pain occurs in the inguinal region, scrotum/labia, and/or femoral triangle. Focal sensory loss over the femoral triangle helps confirm this diagnosis. A local nerve block of the iliohypogastric and ilioinguinal nerves, just medial to the anterosuperior iliac spine, would fail to alleviate symptoms that are from an irritated genitofemoral nerve, which does not pass through this region. However, a paraspinal block of the L1 and L2 spinal nerves, which blocks the genitofemoral nerve (and partially the ilioinguinal and/or iliohypogastric nerves), should relieve the pain.

If a patient with inguinal neuralgia has back pain or no history of previous inguinal or abdominal surgery, then a L1 radiculopathy should be ruled out with magnetic resonance imaging.

8

The Diagnostic Anatomy of the Lumbosacral Plexus

Although traumatic lumbosacral plexopathy is uncommon because the pelvic rim protects this structure, the anatomy and diagnosis of these lesions is still quite underreported. This underreporting in the acute trauma patient is likely related to the following issues: (1) Nerve injury is often ignored while more life-threatening injuries are addressed; (2) orthopedic stabilizations preclude proper examination; (3) many physicians are not familiar with lumbosacral plexus anatomy and diagnosis; (4) mild, and even some moderate, lumbosacral plexus lesions can recover during the weeks to months of acute hospitalization and rehabilitation; and (5) once a residual deficit is noted by the physician, the patient is already transferred out of the trauma ward.

Like other lesions of the nervous system, a prerequisite for proper diagnosis and treatment is mastering the anatomy. As with the brachial plexus, one should have a working knowledge of the major branches of the lumbosacral plexus before attempting to tackle its more proximal anatomical relationships. Discussed in previous sections, the femoral and obturator nerves are the major terminal branches of the lumbar plexus, whereas the sciatic nerve is the main product of the sacral plexus. Fortunately, the lumbosacral plexus does not have as many interconnections, or "cross talk" between neural elements, as does the brachial plexus. The spinal nerve contributions to the lumbosacral plexus do, however, split into anterior and posterior divisions prior to forming terminal branches. Therefore, for learning purposes, the lumbosacral plexus may be artificially separated into four regions: the anterior and posterior lumbar (T12-L4) plexus, and the anterior and posterior sacral (L4-S4) plexus.

♦ The Lumbar Plexus

The lumbar plexus is composed of the T12 to L4 ventral rami, which intercommunicate and coalesce to form anterior and posterior divisions in the substance of the psoas major, anterior to the transverse processes (**Fig. 8–1**). The majority of the lumbar plexus elements are within the psoas muscle. A portion of L4 and all of L5 provide input to the sacral plexus, and not the lumbar plexus.

Overall, terminal branches of the lumbar plexus provide motor and sensory innervation to the lower abdomen, anterior thigh, and medial thigh. Besides a communication with the sacral plexus, there are six branches of significance

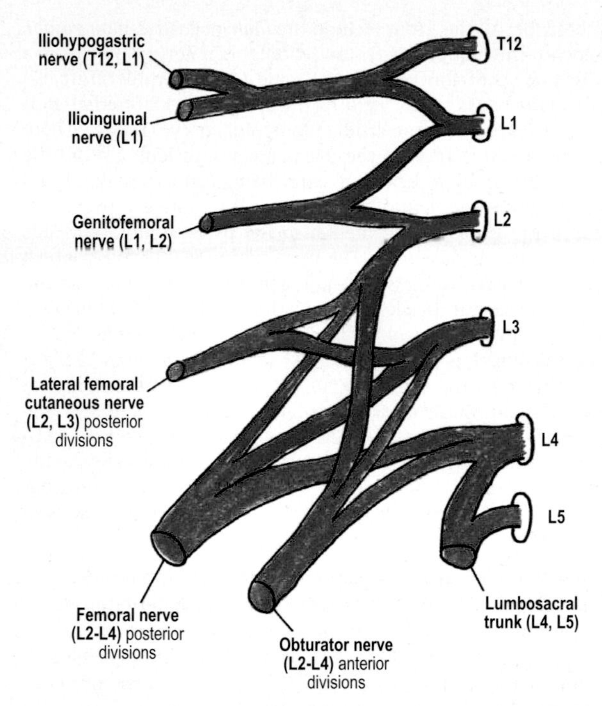

Figure 8–1 Lumbar plexus. The lumbar plexus is composed of the T12 to L4 ventral rami, which intercommunicate and coalesce to form anterior and posterior divisions in the substance of the psoas major, anterior to the transverse processes. A portion of L4, and all of L5, provides input to the sacral plexus, and not the lumbar plexus, via the lumbosacral trunk.

from the lumbar plexus; two groups of three. The first group consists of major branches to the anterior and medial thigh, while the second group includes minor branches to the groin. Both groups, all six branches, constitute the inguinal complex of nerves. The anatomy and function of these branches have been described in a previous chapter.

The three major branches of the lumbar plexus are the *femoral, obturator, and lateral femoral cutaneous nerves*, which arise from the L2, L3, and L4 spinal nerves. Shortly after exiting their respective foramina, these three spinal nerves bifurcate into anterior and posterior divisions. All anterior divisions coalesce to form the obturator nerve; the posterior divisions join to form the femoral nerve. The lateral femoral cutaneous nerve arises from the posterior divisions of L2 and L3 prior to these divisions form the femoral nerve. The most cranial of these three branches, the lateral femoral cutaneous nerve, emerges from the lateral margin of the psoas major and runs around the abdominal wall to the anterosuperior iliac spine, where it exits the pelvis. The femoral nerve runs down and within the posterior aspect of the psoas major, and emerges from between it and the iliacus muscle in the pelvis, approximately 4 cm proximal to the inguinal ligament, from underneath which it enters the thigh. In contrast to the other branches of the lumbar plexus, the obturator nerve runs along the medial aspect of the psoas muscle, emerges from its medial border in the pelvis, and exits into the thigh via the obturator canal.

The three minor branches to the groin include the *iliohypogastric, ilioinguinal, and genitofemoral nerves*. The iliohypogastric and ilioinguinal nerves arise from a common trunk, which has contribution from T12 and L1. This trunk bifurcates within the substance of the psoas major, yielding the more superior (cranial) iliohypogastric nerve (T12,L1) and the more caudal ilioinguinal nerve (only L1), both of which perforate the lateral margin of the psoas major and loop around the abdominal wall toward the inguinal ligament. After being formed by its L1 and L2 spinal nerve contributions, the genitofemoral nerve, alternatively, perforates the *anterior* margin of the psoas major, medial to the psoas minor, and runs caudally on this muscle next to the ureter. The ventral rami of T12 to L2, which contribute to the iliohypogastric, ilioinguinal, and genitofemoral nerves, do not divide into anterior and posterior divisions in the psoas major; this added complexity only occurs in the lower, more major branches of the lumbar plexus.

The lumbosacral trunk, which is made up of a portion of L4 and all of L5 (ventral rami), passes caudally over the sacral ala, adjacent to the sacroiliac joint, to join the sacral plexus. The lumbosacral trunk provides much of the motor and sensory innervation to the common peroneal division of the sciatic nerve. The L4 spinal nerve is known as the *furcal nerve*. Furcal means "forked," and refers to the three proximal divisions of the L4 spinal nerve (ventral ramus only): contribution to the lumbosacral trunk, anterior division to the obturator nerve, and posterior division to the femoral nerve.

- **A few, small motor branches also arise directly from the lumbar plexus. For example, the ventral rami of L1 to L4 provide motor innervation to the quadratus lumborum, and sometimes to the psoas major. Additionally, one or two proximal branches off the femoral nerve also provide motor innervation to the psoas major. When present, the psoas minor is innervated by proximal twigs off the L1 and L2 spinal nerves.**

♦ The Sacral Plexus

The *sacral plexus* is a triangular-shaped complex of neural elements over the inner surface of the sacroiliac joint (**Fig. 8–2**). It is made from the ventral rami of the L4 to S4 spinal nerves, of which S1 to S4 emerge from the ventral sacral foramina. The lumbosacral trunk, made of L4 and L5 contributions to the sacral plexus, passes medial to the obturator nerve, into the lesser pelvis where it joins the sacral plexus. Similar to the lower lumbar plexus, ventral rami contributions to the sacral plexus bifurcate into anterior and posterior divisions prior to forming terminal branches. Nearly all the anterior divisions coalesce to form the tibial division of the sciatic nerve (L4-S3). The posterior divisions, except S3 and S4, form the common peroneal division of the sciatic nerve (L4-S2). The fact that the common peroneal nerve is made of one less division makes sense, considering it is the smaller of the two sciatic nerve components.

In addition to the sciatic nerve, there are several other branches that originate from the sacral plexus, which may be categorized based on whether they originate from the anterior divisions, posterior divisions, or both.

Branches from the Anterior Divisions

Two branches arise from the anterior divisions of the sacral plexus. The first is the *nerve to the quadratus femoris and inferior gemelli*, which arises from the

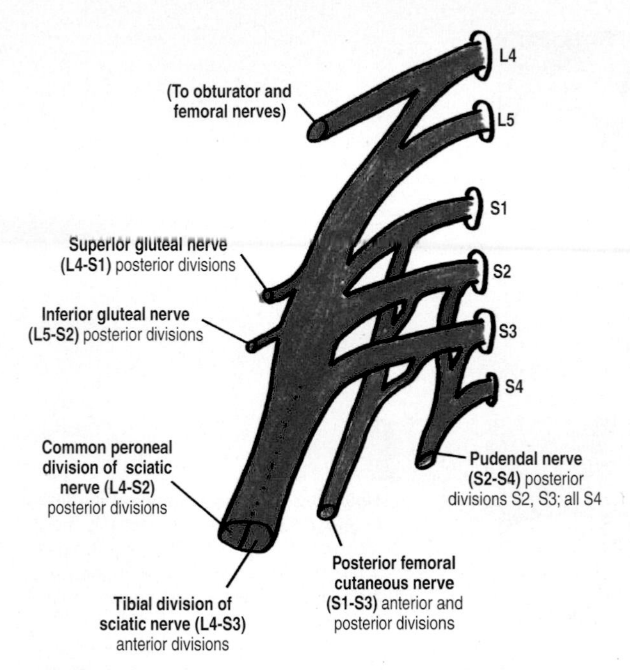

Figure 8–2 Sacral plexus. The sacral plexus is a triangle-shaped complex of neural elements over the inner surface of the sacroiliac joint. It is made from the ventral rami of the L4 to S4 spinal nerves, of which S1 to S4 emerge from the ventral sacral foramina. All spinal nerve contributions, except S4, bifurcate into anterior and posterior divisions (*not shown*) prior to forming terminal branches.

anterior divisions of L4, L5, and S1. The second is the *nerve to the obturator internus and superior gemelli,* which originates from the anterior divisions of L5, S1, and S2. Note that both of these nerves arise from three divisions, however, their origins are shifted by one spinal nerve level. These two nerves provide motor innervation to their named muscles, which together help externally rotate the thigh. Test this movement with the patient seated, legs dangling, while stabilizing the knee with one hand, instruct the patient to resist when you try to pull the lower leg inward (**Fig. 8–3**).

Branches from the Posterior Divisions

There are also two branches from the posterior divisions of the sacral plexus, each similarly originating from three divisions and being shifted by one spinal nerve level. The *superior gluteal nerve* arises from the posterior divisions of L4, L5, and S1, and the *inferior gluteal nerve* from the posterior divisions of L5, S1, and S2.

The superior gluteal nerve exits the pelvis through the greater sciatic foramen above the pyriformis muscle and spreads to innervate the gluteus medius, gluteus minimus, and tensor fascia latae muscles. These three muscles act in conjunction to abduct the thigh. Abduction of an extended thigh (at the hip) is from gluteus medius and minimus contraction. Abduction of a flexed thigh is mostly secondary to tensor fascia latae contraction. To test gluteus thigh abduction, the

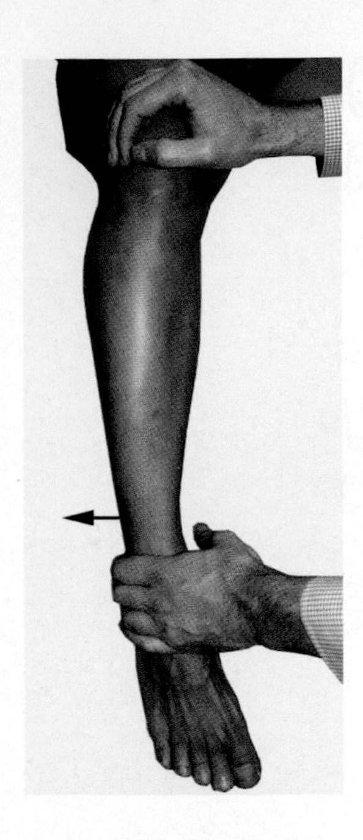

Figure 8–3 External rotation of the flexed thigh (L4-S2) assessment: Test this movement with the patient seated, legs dangling. While stabilizing the knee with one hand, instruct the patient to resist when you pull the lower leg inward.

patient should abduct the thigh against resistance while supine or standing (**Fig. 8–4**). Normally, you should not be able to break thigh abduction. Alternatively,

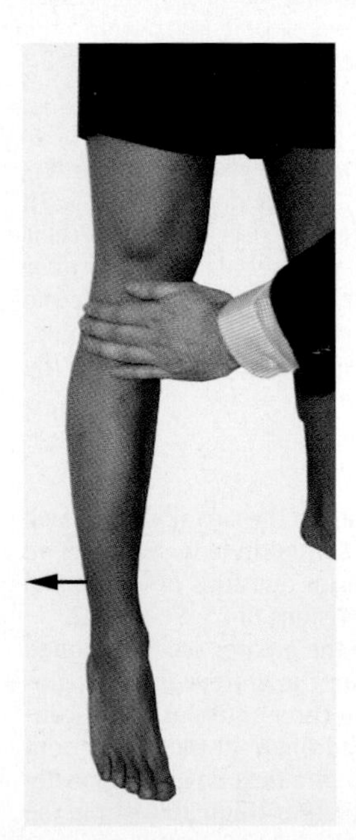

Figure 8–4 Gluteus medius and minimus thigh abduction (L4-S1) assessment: The patient should abduct an extended thigh against resistance while standing (shown) or supine. Normally, you should not be able to break thigh abduction.

to test tensor fascia latae thigh abduction the patient should spread the legs while seated on an examining bench (**Fig. 8–5**).

The inferior gluteal nerve innervates the gluteus maximus muscle, which extends the thigh with some assistance from the hamstrings. The gluteus maximus may be tested in isolation with the patient either prone or standing (**Fig. 8–6**). Start with the leg flexed at the knee to eliminate hamstring substitution, and then instruct the patient to extend the thigh at the hip. Of note, it is normal for this range of motion to be limited. This is because the rectus femoris muscle is placed stretched when the thigh is extended. The buttock may be simultaneously palpated to ascertain muscle contraction.

A Branch from Both the Anterior and Posterior Divisions

The *posterior femoral cutaneous nerve* originates from both the anterior and posterior divisions of S1 to S3. More specifically, it arises from the posterior divisions of S1 and S2, and the anterior divisions of S2 and S3. The posterior femoral cutaneous nerve is also called the *lesser sciatic nerve*, and runs medial and parallel to the sciatic nerve in the buttock region. As both of these "sciatic" nerves pass distally, the posterior femoral cutaneous nerve becomes more superficial and medial, running just lateral to the ischial tuberosity at the lower margin of the gluteus maximus. At the gluteal fold, it pierces the fascia to become subcutaneous. Its sensory territory includes the lower buttock, posterior midline of the thigh, and most of the popliteal region (**Fig. 8–7**). In some individuals, this territory may extend distally to include some posterior calf. Considering their close anatomical relationship, the posterior femoral cutaneous nerve may be damaged along with the proximal sciatic nerve following buttock trauma.

Damage to the posterior femoral cutaneous nerve causes numbness in the lower buttock and posterior thigh, which may be confused with an S2 radiculopathy. These two processes may be differentiated because, in addition to radiating low back pain, patients with an S2 radiculopathy usually have mild gastrocnemius weakness and a depressed ankle reflex.

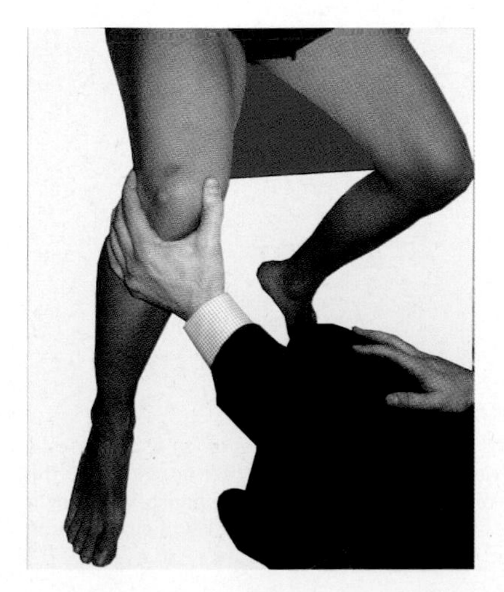

Figure 8–5 Tensor fascia latae thigh abduction (L4-S1) assessment: Have the patient spread the legs while seated on an examining bench. By flexing the hip, contribution to thigh abduction from the gluteal muscles is minimized.

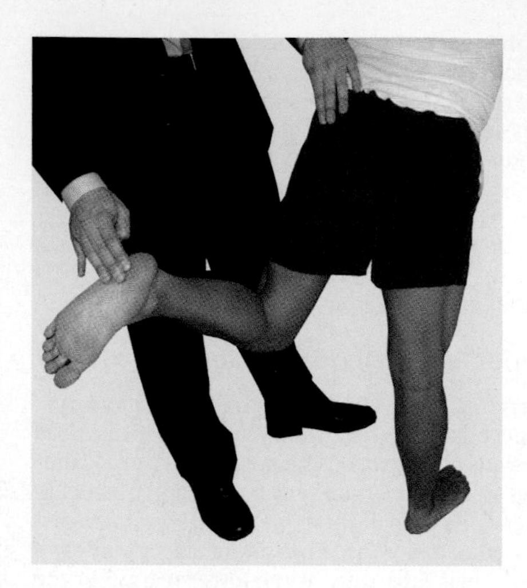

Figure 8–6 Thigh extension (L5-S2) assessment: The gluteus maximus may be tested in isolation with the patient either standing (shown) or prone. Start with the leg flexed at the knee to eliminate hamstring substitution, and then instruct the patient to extend the thigh at the hip. The buttock may be simultaneously palpated to ascertain muscle contraction.

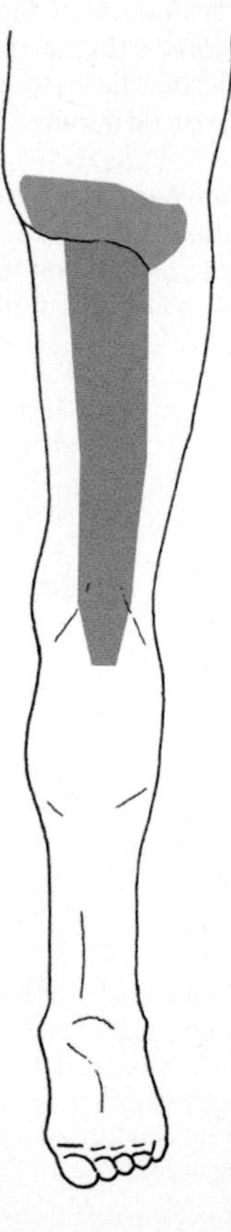

Figure 8–7 Sensory territory of the posterior femoral cutaneous nerve (posterior view). This nerve's sensory territory includes the posterior midline of the thigh, and most of the popliteal region. In some individuals, its territory may extend distally to include some posterior calf.

There are additional, proximal branches from the posterior femoral cutaneous nerve that pierce the fascia and become subcutaneous at the gluteal fold. The more lateral branches are called the *inferior cluneal nerves* and provide sensation to the inferior and lateral buttock. The medial branch is called the *inferior pudendal nerve*, which provides sensation to the scrotum or labia.

Other Branches

The *pudendal nerve* primarily originates from S4, with supplemental input from the anterior divisions of both the S2 and S3 spinal nerves. The pudendal nerve exits the medial aspect of the greater sciatic foramen, turns to enter the lesser sciatic foramen, and makes its way to the pudendal (Alcock's) canal, which is deep to the sacrospinous ligament (**Fig. 8–8**). There are three named branches from the pudendal nerve: (1) the inferior rectal nerve, which innervates the external anal sphincter and skin around the anus, (2) the perineal nerve (the continuation of the pudendal nerve after the inferior rectal nerve branch), which runs with the perineal artery to innervate the posterior scrotum or labia, erectile tissue, and the external urethral sphincter, and (3) the dorsal nerve to the penis or clitoris.

Small branches off the posterior surface of the S1 and S2 ventral rami merge to become the *nerve to the pyriformis*. The pyriformis muscle assists in external rotation of the thigh when flexed (**Fig. 8–3**).

- **As with the brachial plexus, there is variability in the spinal nerve input to the lumbosacral plexus. When T12 provides a large contribution, and S3 only a minimal one, or none at all, the lumbosacral plexus is considered prefixed. In contrast, when T12 provides no input, L1 only a small contribution, and S4 significant input to the plexus (besides the pudendal nerve), the lumbosacral plexus is considered postfixed. Furthermore,**

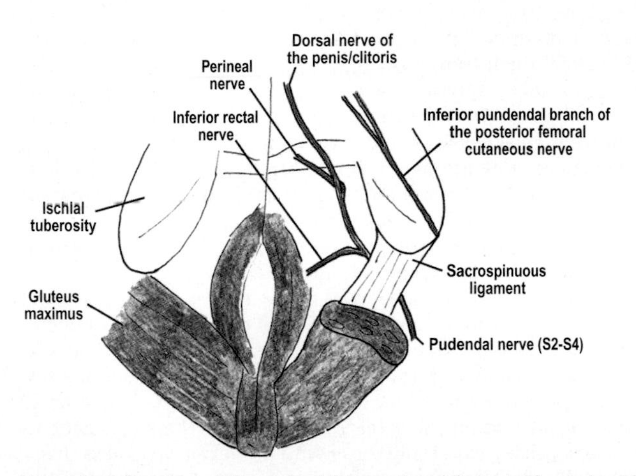

Figure 8–8 Branches of the pudendal nerve (caudal view). The pudendal nerve exits the medial aspect of the greater sciatic foramen, then turns to enter the lesser sciatic foramen, making its way into the pudendal (Alcock's) canal deep to the sacrospinous ligament. There are three branches of the pudendal nerve: the inferior rectal nerve, perineal nerve (the continuation of the pudendal nerves after the inferior rectal nerve branch), and the dorsal nerve to the penis or clitoris.

each branch from the lumbosacral plexus may be composed of additional, or fewer, spinal nerve components than usual.

♦ Diagnostic Approach to the Lumbosacral Plexus

When the pattern of weakness and sensory loss in a lower extremity appears to affect more than one major nerve a lumbosacral plexus lesion should be suspected. The concurrent involvement of certain other plexal branches (i.e., gluteal nerves, posterior cutaneous nerve to the thigh, and/or pudendal nerve) helps confirm this. However, besides these nerves, few other testable nerve branches arise from the lumbosacral plexus, making lesion localization *within* the lumbosacral plexus difficult, and sometimes impossible. The patient's history, risk factors, co-existing injuries, and mechanism of injury provide important information that should be used to help differentiate proximal branch injuries versus true plexal damage. History of a pelvic tumor, radiation, trauma, or complicated delivery is especially pertinent (see below). Aside from motor and sensory deficits found on examination, sympathetic loss, manifesting as erythematous, dry, warm skin, can also be seen with plexal injuries that involve the sympathetic nerves. Radiographic investigations, including plain X-rays, myelography, and CT (computerized tomography) myelography are used to confirm fractures, pseudomeningoceles, hematomas, and foreign bodies, all of which can aid lesion localization. Additionally, electromyography can be quite useful in differentiating plexopathies, proximal mononeuropathies, and radiculopathies.

Lumbar plexus injuries manifest with thigh flexion, thigh adduction, and leg extension weakness. Sensory changes can occur in the lower abdomen (iliohypogastric nerve), groin (ilioinguinal nerve), genitalia/femoral triangle (genitofemoral nerve), lateral thigh (lateral femoral cutaneous nerve), anterior thigh (femoral nerve), medial thigh (femoral and obturator nerves), and medial leg down to the arch of the foot (saphenous nerve). Lumbar or sacral plexus injuries can be partial or complete. The most noticeable deficits with lumbar plexus damage are quadriceps weakness/wasting and anterior thigh sensory loss. For this reason, many patients with lumbar plexus damage are misdiagnosed as having only a femoral neuropathy. Therefore, it is important to remember that for patients with complete or partial femoral palsies, one should check for adductor weakness (obturator nerve) and sensory loss on the anterolateral thigh (lateral femoral cutaneous nerve) to help exclude a lumbar plexus injury.

Sacral plexus damage can cause sciatic nerve motor and sensory loss, sensory loss to the posterior midline thigh (posterior femoral cutaneous nerve), motor loss of the gluteal muscles (superior and inferior gluteal nerves), as well as sexual, bladder, and bowel dysfunction (pudendal nerve, autonomic nervous system). Analogous to the femoral nerve in lumbar plexus injuries, sciatic nerve palsy is the predominant finding in sacral injury patients. Therefore, patients with suspected sciatic palsies, especially those with leg flexion weakness (hamstrings), should be fully evaluated for a sacral plexus injury. Check the patient's sensation in the posterior thigh (posterior femoral cutaneous nerve), thigh abduction and extension (superior and inferior gluteal nerves, respectively), and peri-anal sensation (pudendal nerve damage). Sacral plexus damage is difficult to differentiate from concurrent palsies of the sciatic, inferior gluteal, and posterior cutaneous nerves, all of which can be simultaneously injured distal to the plexus where they together exit the greater sciatic foramen below the pyriformis muscle. The superior gluteal and pudendal nerves exit the pelvis away from these other three nerves; therefore, thigh abduction weakness and perineal sensory loss would be important findings that implicate sacral plexus injury.

Focal damage to the lumbosacral trunk is particularly difficult to diagnose and requires further comment. L5 radiculopathy, lumbosacral trunk damage, sciatic nerve injury predominantly involving the common peroneal division, and common peroneal nerve palsy may all have similar clinical findings, namely a foot drop. A lumbosacral trunk lesion may be differentiated from sciatic or common peroneal palsies because it often causes weakness in the posterior tibialis as well as other more proximal muscles, including the gluteals (thigh extension and abduction). Differentiating an L5 radiculopathy from a lumbosacral trunk lesion is often not possible clinically. Imaging (to rule out nerve root compression) and electrical testing (to document paraspinal muscle denervation) help confirm an L5 radiculopathy. A fracture/dislocation of the ipsilateral sacroiliac joint on CT or X-ray may point toward lumbosacral trunk damage in trauma patients with a foot drop.

Lower sacral plexus (S3-S5) damage causes peri-neal/peri-anal sensory loss, decreased anal sphincter tone, loss of an anal reflex, and loss of a bulbocavernosus reflex. Test the anal reflex (anal wink) by scratching the skin near the anus and observing the sphincter's reflexive contraction. Afferents for this reflex are carried by S5 and efferents by S3-S5. Test the bulbocavernosus reflex by briefly flicking the glans penis while with your other hand you palpate any bulbocavernosus muscle contraction behind the scrotum. Afferents for this reflex are carried by S3 and efferents by S3-S5.

Sympathetic fibers destined for the lower extremity originate from the upper lumbar spinal nerves and enter the sympathetic trunk to be subsequently distributed to the peripheral nerves in the lumbosacral plexus. Therefore, lumbosacral plexus and peripheral nerve (e.g., sciatic nerve) lesions can cause sympathetic abnormalities in the lower extremity (e.g., a warm, dry foot). In contrast, lower lumbar and sacral radiculopathies do not because the injury or compression is proximal to where the sympathetic nerves join the plexus.

Spinal Nerve Dermatomes and Myotomes

Being able to rule out a peripheral nerve problem in patients with presumed spinal radiculopathies is very important, especially in surgical candidates without clear-cut back and radicular pain. In this section, a summary of the respective dermatomes and myotomes for the L1 to S1 spinal nerves is provided. Overall, L2, L3, and L4 radiculopathies should be differentiated from femoral neuropathies, L5 radiculopathy from common peroneal nerve injury, and S1 radiculopathy from a tibial nerve lesion.

The *L1 spinal nerve* provides sensation to the hypogastric area, groin, and base of the penis/mons pubis. Muscle weakness does not occur. Pain within the L1 dermatome is, however, usually non-neural in origin. Local processes, including hernias or lymphadenitis, are often the reason for the pain. Non-neural problems should not cause sensory loss, so if numbness is present, one should strongly consider nerve injury, especially if the patient had previous surgery. Ilioinguinal, iliohypogastric, and genitofemoral neuropathies, as well as upper lumbar plexus lesions, are all in the differential diagnosis of a suspected L1 radiculopathy.

The *L2 spinal nerve* provides sensation to the anterior thigh and motor innervation to the iliopsoas muscles. Therefore, although both a femoral neuropathy and L2 radiculopathy may cause anterior thigh pain, numbness, or paresthesias, their motor deficits are different: femoral neuropathies cause quadriceps weakness; L2 radiculopathies cause iliopsoas weakness. Alternatively, if the motor exam is normal and spine imaging does not reveal a compressive lesion, anterolateral sensory loss on the thigh is probably meralgia paresthetica. For meralgia paresthetica the patellar reflex would be normal.

The *L3 spinal nerve* provides sensation to the lower anterior thigh and knee region, along with motor innervation to the quadriceps and thigh adductors. Therefore, the main differential of an L3 radiculopathy is once again a femoral neuropathy. For patients with a femoral neuropathy, however, adductor strength would be normal, which is not the case for a severe L3 radiculopathy. spine imaging and/or electrodiagnostic testing are required to differentiate an L3 radiculopathy from a lumbar plexus lesion.

The *L4 spinal nerve* carries sensation to the medial leg, in the distribution of the saphenous nerve. It provides substantial motor innervation to the quadriceps via the femoral nerve and the thigh adductors via the obturator nerve. It also provides motor innervation to the anterior tibialis via the common peroneal nerve. To differentiate a femoral neuropathy from a L4 radiculopathy one should check for thigh adductor weakness and foot dorsiflexion weakness, which would only be present with a radiculopathy.

The *L5 spinal nerve* provides sensation to the anterolateral shin, and dorsum of the foot. It also innervates all the muscles innervated by the common peroneal nerve. Therefore, a common peroneal neuropathy should be ruled out in all L5 radiculopathy patients. Fortunately, the L5 nerve root provides motor innervation to other muscles besides those innervated by the common peroneal nerve, including the posterior tibialis and glutei. Therefore, foot inversion (posterior tibialis) should be normal for patients with common peroneal lesions. Of note, many patients with a L5 radiculopathy have depressed or absent ankle jerks. This is because large herniated discs at L4/5 can also partially affect the S1 nerve root.

The *S1 spinal nerve* provides sensation to the lateral aspect (via the sural nerve) and sole (via the plantar nerves) of the foot. Motor innervation includes the muscles of foot plantar flexion, as well as all the foot intrinsics. This pattern of sensory and motor loss closely mimics that of the sciatic nerve's tibial division, and/or the tibial nerve itself. The S1 nerve root, however, also innervates the gluteal muscles via the superior and inferior gluteal nerves. Therefore, in addition to the presence of low back and radicular pain, gluteal weakness helps confirm a S1 radiculopathy. Furthermore, the posterior tibialis (L4, L5; foot inversion) does not receive S1 input, and therefore would be spared with a S1 radiculopathy, but not necessarily for a sciatic or tibial injury. A tibial neuropathy can be differentiated from both a S1 radiculopathy and a proximal sciatic lesion because it would spare both the gluteal muscles and the more proximally innervated hamstrings.

♦ Processes Affecting the Lumbosacral Plexus

As with the brachial plexus, damage to the lumbosacral plexus can be categorized as structural or nonstructural. Structural etiologies include tumors, hemorrhage, postsurgical, obstetric/gynecologic, traumatic, and injections. Nonstructural causes include lumbosacral amyotrophic neuralgia, radiation, vasculitis, diabetes, infection, and hereditary pressure palsies. Some etiologies are discussed further.

Trauma

Traumatic lumbosacral plexopathy is usually partial and is most commonly caused by high-speed deceleration (i.e., motor vehicle) accidents where the pelvis or hip is fractured/dislocated. In fact, about one quarter of all pelvic fractures are associated with nerve damage, plexal or otherwise. Most traumatic lumbosacral plexus injuries are postganglionic from stretch or traction; however, sacroiliac joint fractures or dislocations may cause spinal nerve avulsion. These avulsions may occur in or out of the spinal canal. As in the cervical region, myelography and MR imaging assists in the diagnosis of nerve avulsion by documenting pseudomeningoceles. Considering the proximity of the lumbosacral trunk to the sacroiliac joint, it may be selectively damaged with fracture/dislocations in this area. Because the lumbosacral trunk carries many fibers destined for the common peroneal division of the sciatic nerve, these patients present with a foot drop.

Traumatic or iatrogenic injury of the lumbosacral plexus may be divided into four diagnostic zones, with most patients having more then one zone either completely or partially involved. Zone 1 involves the anterior divisions of the lumbar plexus (the obturator nerve, medial thigh). Zone 2 involves the posterior divisions of the lumbar plexus (the femoral and lateral femoral cutaneous nerves, anterior, medial, and lateral thigh/leg). Zone 3 refers to the anterior divisions of the sacral plexus (the tibial division of the sciatic nerve). Zone 4 involves the posterior divisions of the sacral plexus (the common peroneal division of the sciatic nerve as well as the superior and inferior gluteal nerves). The utility of this zone-based categorization of lumbosacral injuries may prove to be limited because most injuries do not follow these convenient boundaries. Preliminary data reveals that trauma most frequently involves either the sacral plexus alone, or the complete lumbosacral plexus. Isolated, traumatic lumbar plexus injuries are quite rare.

Retroperitoneal Hemorrhage

Patients with hemophilia or taking anticoagulation medications may have spontaneous retroperitoneal hemorrhages. Patients with normal clotting may also have retroperitoneal bleeds following trauma, retroperitoneal surgery, or groin catheterization. Hemorrhage may be confined to the psoas muscle, iliacus muscle, or abdominal wall; larger hemorrhages may involve all three of these areas. A psoas muscle hemorrhage would selectively compress the lumbar plexus. These patients have acute, often severe, back pain radiating to their groin and anterior thigh. Weakness occurs in the quadriceps, iliopsoas, and occasionally the thigh adductors. Severe pain may limit the accuracy of the neurological assessment. Sensory loss in a lumbar plexus distribution, mostly in the groin and anterior thigh, may occur. Hip movement is painful and patients are often most comfortable with the thigh flexed at the hip.

More-extensive hemorrhages affecting the lumbar plexus can tract caudally to also compress the lumbosacral trunk and sacral plexus. Alternatively, focal hemorrhages in the iliacus muscle (i.e., iliacus compartment), which typically can occur following groin catheterization, may selectively compress the femoral nerve.

Lumbosacral Plexitis (Amyotrophic Neuralgia)

This clinical ailment of uncertain etiology affects both lumbosacral plexus as it does the brachial plexus. Patients present with an acute or subacute onset of proximal lower-extremity pain, often radiating down the anteromedial or posterior thigh, sometimes down into the lower leg. The pain is quite severe and limits motor assessment. Days to weeks later (on average 1 week), weakness appears in the distribution of the pain. Paresthesias may also occur. Plexal involvement is usually partial, affecting either multiple plexal branches, or just one (e.g., the femoral nerve). Over time, the pain and weakness slowly resolve, with many patients having *close to* complete resolution after several months.

Proximal Diabetic Neuropathy

Weakness is the predominant manifestation of proximal diabetic neuropathy (diabetic amyotrophy). It usually causes thigh flexion, thigh adduction, thigh abduction, and leg extension weakness (femoral, obturator, and gluteal nerves). Atrophy of the proximal thigh and hip girdle may occur. Although pain can be severe, concentrated in the back, groin, or anteromedial thigh, many patients have only mild or no pain. As with idiopathic lumbosacral plexitis, weakness and pain from proximal diabetic neuropathy usually resolves in several months (3 to 18). Residual stiffness and weakness can remain, however. Acute diabetic neuropathies only affecting the femoral nerve are quite rare; most patients actually have other, perhaps subtle, involvement of the lumbar plexus. The etiology of proximal diabetic neuropathy may be epineurial microvasculitis.

Two distinct types of proximal diabetic neuropathy can occur. The first type is descriptively called *proximal asymmetric neuropathy*. Patients with this type have abrupt onset of unilateral weakness as well as a severe amount of inguinal and thigh pain. Patients report trouble ambulating because of knee buckling. Diabetic patients with this type usually do not have peripheral (stocking-glove) neuropathy, and are not usually insulin dependent. A history of recent weight loss, curiously, is often present.

The second type is called *proximal symmetrical neuropathy*, and often occurs in insulin dependent diabetics with a history of peripheral (stocking-glove) neuropathy. The onset of weakness is slow, manifesting over days to weeks. The weakness is bilateral, although still asymmetrical. Pain can occur, but is also slow in onset.

Neoplastic and Radiation Damage

Pelvic tumors may cause plexopathy, and in these patients, severe pain, not weakness, is the primary complaint. The initial presentation is usually an insidious onset of back or pelvic pain that radiates to the thigh or leg. Weakness and/or numbness can occur, but these deficits are usually minimal. If the tumor involves the most caudal fibers of the sacral plexus bilaterally, incontinence can also occur. Primary tumors affecting the lumbosacral plexus include colorectal, uterine, prostate, and ovarian. Secondary, or metastatic, tumors involving the lumbosacral plexus include breast, sarcoma, lymphoma, testicular, and thyroid. Malignant invasion of the lumbosacral plexus has four patterns: lumbosacral involvement only, sacral plexus involvement only, complete ipsilateral lumbosacral plexus involvement, and bilateral lower sacral involvement.

Pelvic, or lower paraspinal, radiation therapy may cause lumbosacral plexopathy. Radiation doses greater than 5000 rads are usually required, with symptoms appearing slowly, on average 5 years later (range 1 to 30 years). Radiation plexopathy is usually painless, or with minimal pain, which is a key finding that helps differentiate radiation plexopathy from recurrent tumor, which is usually painful. Radiation plexopathy presents with an insidious onset of weakness. The rate of progression and completeness of the lesion are variable. The majority of cases are bilateral. Numbness and paresthesias may occur. Weakness usually stabilizes only after it is already profound. Improvement is unlikely. Myokymic discharges on needle electromyography occur in radiation plexopathy, being a useful way to help exclude recurrent tumor.

Index

Note: Page numbers followed by f and t indicate figures and tables, respectively.

B

C

D

E

F

G

H

I

K

L

M

N

O

P

Q

R

S

T

U

V